# A DAY'S JOURNEY

## STORIES OF HOPE AND DEATH-DEFYING JOY

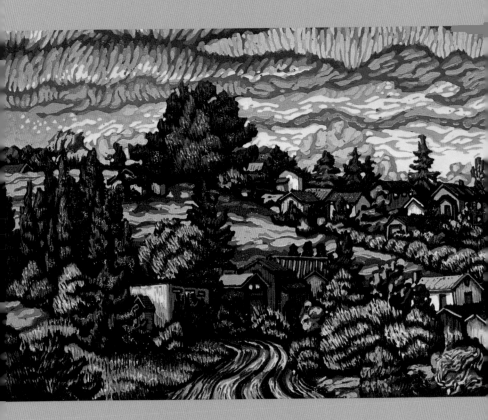

# TIM KEESEE

FOREWORD BY JONI EARECKSON TADA

"As Keesee has reported news of the gospel's advance from the frontlines, in this latest missive he describes how Jesus meets us on the frontlines of our suffering. Proverbs tells us that the sweetness of a friend comes from his earnest counsel. *A Day's Journey* chronicles the profoundly sweet way that Jesus uses friendship to bless and strengthen us in our deepest pain."

Gloria Furman, co-editor of *Word-Filled Women's Ministry* and author of *Labor with Hope*

"I know Tim Keesee as a storyteller—a man who has committed much of his life to seeking, finding, and telling stories about the ways God is at work in and through His people as they labor at the frontiers of world missions. But a recent diagnosis of terminal cancer has inspired him to tell new stories—stories of his own life and stories from the lives of other people who exhibit unshakeable hope and death-defying joy. Beautifully written and inspiringly grounded in the deepest truths, this is a book that will give strength and courage to all who are making their way through uncertain times and difficult days."

Tim Challies, author of *Seasons of Sorrow*

"Cancer. My wife, myself, and now my daughter. Five years— three battles. Tim's battling too. With his wonderfully gifted pen, he's brought us along on the journey, filling each page with stories of fierce faith in the face of suffering. I needed this book. You do too. Take and read."

Mitch Maher, lead pastor, Redeemer Community Church in Katy, Texas; creator, presenter, *Clarifying the Bible*

"The first time I read something from Tim Keesee, I was captivated by his writing. I still am. Tim's worldview arrests my heart and my mind. I love his love for the Lord, and the sobriety with which he shepherds God's people and the Father's relentless truth. You may be tempted to sample this book as you would the cashews in a pretty dish on someone's coffee table. Don't do this. Dig in. Soak in his wisdom. Be taken by truth, perhaps as never before. The time you spend here will be a worthy investment. I promise."

Robert Wolgemuth, bestselling author

"Cancer is the reality check that no one wants. Uncertainties, fears, pain, relentless grief—Tim draws them close through life stories, then shines a searchlight on God's steadfast love, our refuge and true reality. *A Day's Journey* brings strange comfort to my own fearful, hopeful journey. I'm in good company."

Karen Hubbard, friend and fellow cancer survivor

"I've traveled with my friend Tim to some dangerous destinations for gospel advance. Now on a different kind of journey—the terra incognita of cancer—I've been watching him scrutinize Scripture and lean hard into Christ. This book is a blazing torch to guide us through the shadowlands."

Dr. David Hosaflook, missionary

# A DAY'S JOURNEY

# A DAY'S JOURNEY

## STORIES OF HOPE AND DEATH-DEFYING JOY

# TIM KEESEE

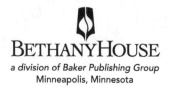

BETHANYHOUSE

*a division of Baker Publishing Group*
Minneapolis, Minnesota

Published by Bethany House Publishers
Minneapolis, Minnesota
www.bethanyhouse.com

Bethany House Publishers is a division of
Baker Publishing Group, Grand Rapids, Michigan

Printed in the United States of America

Library of Congress Control Number: 2023018334
ISBN 978-0-7642-4174-1 (paperback)
ISBN 978-0-7642-4230-4 (casebound)
ISBN 978-1-4934-4383-3 (ebook)

The author is represented by the literary agency of Wolgemuth & Associates.

Baker Publishing Group publications use paper produced from sustainable forestry practices and post-consumer waste whenever possible.

23  24  25  26  27  28  29      7  6  5  4  3  2  1

To Sarah and Tim—
our arrows sent
with love

# CONTENTS

Foreword by Joni Eareckson Tada    13

A Word of Thanks    17

Readers' Guide    19

**SETTING OUT**

Dear Diary    27

One Day to Live    39

Stumbling into the Future    49

Time in a Rectangle    57

**ALONG THE WAY**

In the Eye of a Storm    67

Day of Hopeful Planting    81

Knee-Deep in Wonders    95

The Day the Walls Came Down    107

Brave Music    121

The Sweet Psalmist of Texas    141

Five Witnesses    151

## TOWARD EVENING

Another Way to Die    165

In Habakkuk's Tower    169

Chemo Days    179

Christmas Day    197

Numbered Days    203

All My Days    225

Notes    229

It is [God] to whom and with whom we travel, and while he is the End of our journey, he is also at every stopping place.[1]

—Elisabeth Elliot, *All That Was Ever Ours*

# FOREWORD

## Before You Begin

Quadriplegia taxes my breathing, so I was winded after giving my speech at the Ligonier Conference. But there was no time to recoup. I had to race to an interview across the massive church campus. I wheeled to an exit but saw steps on the other side. Glancing this way and that, I fumed. *There must be a door with a ramp somewhere.*

I found one and zipped outside. Halfway down a long walkway, I sensed a man running to keep up with me. When we arrived at another set of steps, my heart sank. Lost in a labyrinth of walkways and stairs, I gave the man a bewildered look. Maybe he was a groundskeeper who knew the way.

"Quick, follow me!" he said, and within minutes we reached the correct building and made a dash for the media room. My new friend wasn't about to leave my side until I reached our destination. *Who is this amazing guy?* I wondered.

It was my first encounter with Tim Keesee. Although a presenter at the conference with his own busy schedule, he had dropped everything to help a disabled woman in distress. That's the way Tim is wired. He gladly participates in the hardships of others.

Just watch his DVD series, *Dispatches from the Front*. You'll find Tim laboring alongside Thai Christians risking their lives to rescue women out of slavery. He's bushwhacking his way through a jungle, helping to carry supplies to a church outpost. He's crouching with his journal by a charcoal fire alongside a handful of Africans, scribbling down their faith stories by firelight. Back in his tent, he takes out his pen and fills more pages. He is tireless. Relentless. And utterly dedicated to his quest. Tim is out to capture unheard-of examples of Spirit-inspired courage.

There's a reason for his quest.

Tim knows that with every hard effort bravely faced, with every gentle word spoken under affliction, and with every cross cheerfully shouldered, the Church is ratcheted up to a higher level. When sufferers exalt their Savior, they infuse iron into the faith of others. Their testimonies endow people with a clearer view of God. And all of it makes the body of Christ strong and purehearted. The Church—especially the Western Church—is in urgent need of such examples.

Tim Keesee is not slowing down his quest. Once again, he's been hard at work cataloguing the stories of courageous Christians. But this time, his journal looks different. In *A Day's Journey*, he not only records the faith stories of others . . . he includes his own. Tim's recent battle against a fierce cancer has enlisted him among his brave examples. And we, his readers, are all the richer for it.

*A Day's Journey* was written for you. The stories on the following pages are compiled for the enrichment of your faith. For when it comes to hardships, we *all* need hope, help, and a little guidance. Titus 2:7 (NIV) says, "In everything set them an example by doing what is good," and with every chapter, Tim provides convincing examples of how to do what is good—that is, how to endure the weightiest of afflictions with an eye to God's glory.

So, as a fellow sufferer, I commend this excellent volume to you. Picture yourself in its pages. Linger over each story and ask your soul questions. Inquire of your heart as to the depth of its confidence in Christ. Poke your finger into your faith to test its resilience.

Better yet, pull out a journal and do what Tim has been doing for years—take notes and learn from those who consider their afflictions as light and momentary compared to an eternal weight of glory.

Joni Eareckson Tada

Joni and Friends International Disability Center

# A WORD OF THANKS

In the last chapter of Romans, Paul mentions nearly forty individuals who had an impact on his ministry—saints with whom he had shared the risks and friendships of Gospel work. I love that chapter for the *esprit de corps* it embodies among fellow soldiers of Jesus Christ. This bit of the book is my Romans 16 postscript.

Much of *A Day's Journey* was written while I was undergoing treatments related to my ongoing battle with cancer. Consequently, I want to give special thanks to my oncologist, Dr. Saeeda Chowdhury. From the time she took me as her patient, she brought her care, skill, and tenacity to this fight—day or night. I also owe deep gratitude to all the nurses and doctors at the Blood and Marrow Transplant Unit at Greenville Memorial Hospital, especially Susan Funk and Dr. Suzanne Fanning.

Other doctors' counsel was also inestimable—Dr. Rachel Hansen of Changchun, China, and Dr. Andy Sanders and Dr. Don Townsend, both of Augusta, Georgia. I often describe cancer in traveling terms—a journey or a path—but some places have been more like a labyrinth with no clear way forward. These three physicians were part of my Good Shepherd's leading at critical times.

While I was battling cancer and writing this book, there were more people than I could possibly name here who were praying, pitching in to help where they could, and sending timely letters that gave me fresh courage. So many dear friends were like Aaron and Hur for me, and while I know I will miss some, I'd like to name a few: Kevin and Leslie Cathey; Steve Leatherwood; Bert Arrowood; Allan Sherer; Roger Weil; Ben Henning; Dave Hutton; Rosaria Butterfield; Julie Zickefoose; my cousin Renee Marsh; my pastor Peter Hubbard and his wife, Karen; David Hosaflook; J.D. Crowley; Elisa Chodan; John Piper; Joni Eareckson Tada; and my young friend Zoe Farmer.

The Frontline Missions team—both home office and worldwide—loved us like family. I especially want to thank John Hutcheson for all the miles we've traveled together and especially all the time you spent the past two years covering speaking engagements for me; Ben Ebner for your steady and strong leadership, which kept the whole team steady and strong; and Ronny Marmol for your faithful friendship and for investing your time in helping me regain strength to travel again. I am also humbled by the love that was extended to us from Frontline's families overseas and from little house churches scattered from North Africa to northern China. What an encouragement that prayers ascended on our behalf in Arabic and Albanian, in Ukrainian, Hindi, Uzbek, Mandarin, Tagalog, and Bahasa!

On the publishing side of turning my journals into the book you hold, special thanks go to two Andrews: Andrew Wolgemuth of Wolgemuth & Associates was superb and ever ready to help, and Andy McGuire, my acquisitions editor at Bethany House Publishers, who was a delight to work with. I'm also grateful to Elisa Haugen—editor extraordinaire—for working through my journals with me.

Finally, and foremost, Debbie—I could never have made it this far without you!

# READERS' GUIDE

Three miles an hour. For most of history, that walking pace has been the speed at which much of humanity moved. Sure, there were camels and horses, and Hannibal's army famously used elephants to get around. However, four legs instead of two were used mostly for battles or as beasts of burden. The average person got around the old-fashioned way, and travelers in ancient times measured their distance by how far they could go in a day at walking speed. They would simply say they went "a day's journey," which was approximately twenty-five miles. Of course, *a day's journey* wasn't a precise measure because many things affected it—such as terrain, risks encountered, weather, as well as the locations of early versions of a motel.

This book is about days. It's about how we spend them and (like those early trekkers) about the twists and turns we encounter along the way. So I took this ancient measure as my title: *A Day's Journey*. When I originally envisioned this book, it was to be similar to my previous books and films in the *Dispatches from the Front* series—travelogues written from distant outposts of Christ's Kingdom. Only *this* book would not be written from just one country but would be a global odyssey with stories of one great blood-bought family gathered from many nations. It would be a preview of Revelation 5:9 between two covers:

> And they sang a new song, saying,
> "Worthy are you to take the scroll
>     and to open its seals,
> for you were slain, and by your blood you ransomed
>         people for God
>     from every tribe and language and people and
>         nation."

I couldn't wait to get started filling my journal with stories of this every-tribe-every-tongue Gospel! But then something happened. To repurpose Emily Dickinson's lines,

> Because I could not stop for Death,
> He kindly stopped for me.[1]

*Cancer* stopped for me. People deal with their suffering in different ways. For me—I write. So, bound by weakness, chemo, and oncologist appointments, this book became a more personal dispatch written from the cancer front. Although I have been in this battle for three years now, I know that what I have experienced and suffered cannot be compared to what others suffer. Since I began this book, at least a dozen close friends have died from a variety of causes. Others suffer from severe chronic illnesses that are too heavy to bear—and yet they do. And others carry the unyielding pain of sorrow over an untimely grave or the utter helplessness of watching dementia erase a loved one's ties to the past, the present, and those who care for them the most. As I have faced cancer, many of these hurting people have reached out to assure me of their prayers and understanding. I am humbled by their stories of hope and endurance and am grateful for all the ways they have pointed me to Christ so I could look up and sing:

O Lord, my Rock and my Redeemer
Strong defender of my weary heart
My sword to fight the cruel deceiver
And my shield against his hateful darts
My song when enemies surround me
My hope when tides of sorrow rise
My joy when trials are abounding
Your faithfulness, my refuge in the night.[2]

To aid my fellow travelers through this book, I've set up milestones along the way by dividing *A Day's Journey* into three parts:

Setting Out
Along the Way
Toward Evening

Every traveler (and reader) has to answer this big question: Where am I going? And so, in "Setting Out," I have written a few essays about time, its swiftness and surprises, about the power of memory and the value of days—including the ordinary and seemingly uninteresting ones, like you are probably having right now. On their own, such days may not be very impressive, but taken all together they are a string of pearls!

The last section, "Toward Evening," is excerpts from my journal written on my cancer journey as I have walked this tortuous path. I pray that these entries scribbled during chemo infusions and sleepless nights will strengthen the hearts of the hurting and magnify Jesus, our sure Hope.

"Setting Out" is the early morning hours of the journey with the sun at your back, while the final section, "Toward Evening," is when the day is drawing down and golden light breaks between the lengthening shadows.

At the heart of this book is "Along the Way." This section is filled with stories of people who have taught me so much about courage, hope, joy, wonder, compassion, and a deeper understanding of the Gospel. I spent a day with each of them and wrote their stories. The writer of Hebrews had such saints in mind when he wrote that we are to be "imitators of those who through faith and patience inherit the promises" (Hebrews 6:12). I've seen the ways they work and worship, the ways they pray and sing, the ways they love their neighbors and the ways they love their enemies—even when beaten black and blue for the sake of Christ. In seeing how they number *their* days, I've learned better how to spend *mine*.

All of these days are written in the moment, capturing as much life as possible in the beautiful ordinary of a day. The historian David McCullough tells a wonderful story about the painter John Singer Sargent, who was the foremost portraitist of his time. In 1903, Sargent was commissioned to paint the official portrait of President Theodore Roosevelt. Sargent spent several days at the White House sizing up the setting and, above all, trying to get a word in with the energetic young president as to when they could do the portrait session. McCullough relates what happened next:

> One morning the two met unexpectedly as Roosevelt was descending the stairway.
>
> When might there be a convenient time for the president to pose for him, Sargent asked.
>
> "Now!" said the president.
>
> So there he is in the painting, standing at the foot of the stairs, his hand on the newel post. It is a great portrait, capturing more of the subtleties of the Roosevelt personality than any ever done of him.
>
> And it's a good story. Moments come and go, the president was telling the painter. Here is the time, seize it, do your best.[3]

I am deeply grateful to those who opened their doors to me to let me meet them at the foot of their staircase, so to speak, and paint a portrait of their day. These days are not filtered, photoshopped images of their lives but instead ones that show life with all its pressing demands and unanswered questions, so that the silver thread of God's grace might be seen all the more as it runs through the routines of their days.

Some of the people whose days unfold here are well-known. Others you haven't heard of before but, like I am, you will be glad you met them. All of them have things to teach us about how we will spend the precious bits of our vapor life—the endurance we need, the joy we have, the Gospel we love, the Cross we bear, and the hope we embrace until faith becomes sight.

As I set out to write this book, capturing in my journal the struggles with living and dying, I have feared at times that I would not finish this book. I've known in full measure the admixtures of sorrow and pain that come from spotted scans, unrelenting nausea, and days of bone-burrowing fatigue. So my fear was not unfounded, and I understand novelist Ann Patchett's response to a brush with death when she wrote, "Were I to die, I'd be taking the entire world of my novel with me—no significant loss to literature, sure, but the thought of losing all the souls inside me was unbearable. Those people were my responsibility."[4] She would have lost her fictional characters, but I would lose the stories of friends—family stories of brothers and sisters who are the pride and joy of their Father.

This narrowing path I walk has more readily reminded me that I "have this treasure in jars of clay, to show that the surpassing power belongs to God and not to us" and that "this light momentary affliction is preparing for us an eternal weight of glory beyond all comparison" (2 Corinthians 4:7, 17). I really am discovering more of His strength in my weakness. Still, though, I know my discoveries are only like wading into the surf of a boundless ocean. By grace, these are the dispatches I've been able to scribble out as I've walked these days. Here toward the evening of my journey, the light has not faded, and I welcome your company.

23

# SETTING OUT

Satisfy us in the morning with your steadfast love,
that we may rejoice and be glad all our days.

—Psalm 90:14

# DEAR DIARY

To-day is always commonplace; it is yesterday that is beautiful, and to-morrow that is full of possibilities. . . . We admit the meaning of life taken altogether, but it is very hard to break up that recognition into fragments, and to feel the worth of these fleeting moments which, just because they are here, seem to be of small account.[1]

—Alexander Maclaren, from the sermon
"Redeeming the Time"

Kmart was the shopping mecca of my small town, although it was a rarity for me to step inside this discount world of wonders. Likely I was there that day to buy shoes for the new school year, as the necessity of my physical presence was the only reason Mama would bring an eleven-year-old along with her to shop. As I walked through the store, suddenly there it was on the clearance table: my beginnings as a writer. It was a five-year diary with a leatherette cover embossed with a lion— the kind of lion a knight would be proud to have emblazoned on his shield. The diary also had an intricate brass latch with a key hanging by a thread. This real brass lock would secure my future secrets from the prying eyes and fingers of my big brother and baby sisters. And all for a mere twenty-five cents. Even on a grass cutter's income, I could swing this!

I rediscovered my first diary in a box rescued from the attic of my parents' house when the place was sold. The old journal was mixed in with plastic army men, faded ribbons from track events, and some superhero bubble gum cards. As I reread the entries, I certainly did not see the glints of a child prodigy—it was about what you would expect from a kid's diary—but the best part was that I kept writing in it. And for over fifty years now, I've continued to keep journals. I now have a shelf full of them—and more stuffed in boxes. Their ink and coffee-stained pages sketch miniatures of people—many long since gone— whose laughter, wisdom, and affection filled my life, and the overflow inked the pages of my journals. Some of my journals capture crossroad decisions, while other journals record distant journeys. It's a happy convergence that *journey* and *journal* have the same French root: *jour*, which means "day." So, a journey is the measure of a day, and a journal is a daily record of life and our encounters with people and places.

To me, the journals by which all other travel journals are inevitably—and often unfavorably—compared are *The Journals of Lewis and Clark*. I share historian Stephen Ambrose's enthusiasm:

> Lewis and Clark's exploration of the western two thirds of the continent was our epic voyage, their account of it is our epic poem. Sitting before the nightly campfire, using a quill pen that had to be dipped into the inkwell every other word, balancing their leather-covered journals on their knees, Captains Meriwether Lewis and William Clark described the day's events, as well as the land and its people and its flora and fauna, in a prose remarkable for its verve, sharp imagery, tension, and immediacy.
>
> Reading the journals puts you in the canoe with them. . . . You and the captains are in a constant state of surprise, because

as you read, and as they write, you never know what's around the bend of the river, or what will happen next.[2]

Lewis and Clark's journals *made* history, but for us lesser mortals, our journals will not be studied or celebrated centuries from now. Yet, our daily writings still do something important: They capture the beautiful rhythms of ordinary life. And most days of our rather obscure lives *are* ordinary, and that's what I appreciate about the journals of Charles Loeber. His diaries are not housed in the Library of Congress—instead, they are in a cigar box on my bookshelf.

Many years ago, three of Loeber's pocket diaries came to me in a box of his papers that no one else at the auction wanted. His little journals were from the years 1900, 1901, and 1902. I don't know anything about him beyond what was in the box, but at the turn of the century, he was a draftsman in an entry-level engineering job. He was a conscientious, church-going young man, who kept a few close friends and was careful with his money. Even his small handwriting seemed to be an act of economy. Among his resolutions for the new year 1901 was "Save $100."

Loeber's weeks had a quiet rhythm to them. He noted the books he read and the friends he visited. He occasionally wrote "Rain" at the top of the page. He saw a lunar eclipse once, and he recorded the news of President McKinley's assassination. On Sundays, Loeber captured the highlights of the sermon in his diary, and after church he usually walked a young lady, named Minnie Mae, home.

My favorite part of Charles Loeber's journal, though, is how hundreds of times he summarized his day with "Business as usual." Day after day, week after week, "Business as usual" crowned most entries. Loeber would go on to become a successful engineer—building schools, hospitals, and churches in China, Korea, and America. Despite his achievements, if later in life he kept a diary, I somehow expect he still wrote "Business as usual" above most days.

Loeber's habitual headline is a reminder that most days *are* ordinary. Ordinary days change with the seasons of life and, of course, from person to person. But for all of us, our routine ruts, our business-as-usual days are the stuff of life.

My day usually slow-starts after sunrise. I've always thought getting up before the sun does is rushing things—and rushing is not something I do first thing in the morning. A simple breakfast and coffee get me started. Coffee in hand, I settle in with my Bible for my morning reading and prayer. Murphy the Cat slips onto my lap and makes for a warm, furry prop for my Bible. Occasionally his big green eyes peer into mine before he settles in again.

The rest of the morning is spent at the mission office—in meetings, answering correspondence, etc. My wife, Debbie, has been my assistant and chief organizing officer for years. She

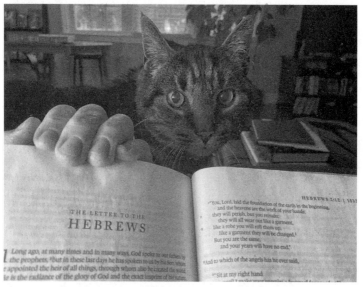

Morning with Murphy

juggles a lot as she fields questions on the phone and in the in-box—and always makes me look better than I deserve. We head home for a quick lunch. Then Debbie may start some laundry before heading back to the office, while I settle in on the back porch with coffee and cat for an afternoon of writing—maybe an article or, in this case, this chapter.

Ink on paper is how I compose—and I'm very particular about the ink, the pen that houses it, and the paper that it's spread on. For years, I've carried a Parker rollerball in my pocket. My sturdy Parker is always at the ready, except when I'm in high deserts, where the ink gets dry and scratchy and I resort to a pencil. I know I'm an anachronism, but I know I'm not alone, as novelist Mark Helprin concurs:

> There is magic in writing by hand: the pauses; sometimes the racing; the scratching out; the closeness of the eyes to the page. . . . A pen (somehow) helps you think and feel. And although once you find a pen you like you'll probably stick with it the way an addict sticks with heroin, it can be anything from a Mont Blanc to a Bic. The same for paper. There are beautiful, smooth, heavy papers, but great works have been written on ration cards, legal pads and the kind of cheap paper they sell in developing countries—grayish white, almost furry, with flecks of brown and black that probably came from lizards and bats that jumped in the paper makers' vats.[3]

Speaking of furry, Murphy scrunches up closer to the porch screen for a better view of the bird feeder. Today the feeder and the trees resemble the airspace over O'Hare, aswirl with cardinals and blue jays, towhees and titmice, chickadees and nuthatches, thrashers and doves. Occasionally a swarm of grackles will swoop in and scatter them all. I really like these bad boys of the backyard as they strut around like pirates. They're as black and glistening as an oil slick and have lemon-yellow eyes that don't miss a thing. Grackles have a coarse squawk that sounds like they burn through a pack a day. They squawk at the other birds, at each other, and sometimes at me. They are delightfully cranky. When they tire of their little game—a bird version of king of the hill—they are off in a flash of feathers and catcalls.

Murphy is unmoved by all of this—probably because he's now asleep. The late afternoon sun is warming me to the idea of a nap as well. If I nap now, perhaps I'll be sharp enough to read and write late into the evening as I used to do. It's only a short debate with myself before I slip into a deep sleep, while sitting up amid a scattering of books and papers with pen in hand, because profound fatigue weighs on me every waking moment. I'm thankful to still have enough strength to push through my day until I hit the inevitable wall—but the wall seems to be moving closer.

I'm writing of my typical day, but the reality is cancer has forever altered my days. The strength and expanse of a normal day for me just a year or two back are out of reach now. My smaller days are wedged into a calendar filled with doctor appointments, infusions, blood draws, scans, and biopsies.

Value the ordinary days because they can suddenly change. Living for the weekend, waiting for that next breakthrough that will finally bring happiness, or wanting to speed up the clock are all sure ways of trampling precious bits of life in the rush to be somewhere else. Sometimes we are forced to look back and see what we've missed. That's the point Aleksandr Solzhenitsyn makes in his semi-biographical novel *Cancer Ward*, which is based on his experiences as a cancer patient in a Soviet hospital. His stories draw on the diverse lives of patients who are suddenly brought together in one confining place because of one life-altering disease.

Dr. Dontsova, the lead doctor in Solzhenitsyn's story, is a compassionate physician toughened by thirty years of dealing with death. Dontsova viewed all her patients and their pathologies in cold textbook terms. But in a terrible role reversal, she discovers she has a malignant tumor. Solzhenitsyn writes:

> Then suddenly, within a few days, her own body had fallen out of this great, orderly system. It had struck the hard earth and was now like a helpless sack crammed with organs—organs which might at any moment be seized with pain and cry out. . . .
> Her world had capsized, the entire arrangement of her existence was disrupted. She was not yet dead, and yet she had had to give up her husband, her son, her daughter, her grandson, and her medical work as well, even though it was her own work, medicine, that would now be rolling over her and through her like a noisy train. In a single day she had to give up everything and suffer, a pale-green shadow, not knowing for a long time whether she was to die irrevocably or return to life.
> It had once occurred to her that there was a lack of color, joy, festivity in her life—it was all work and worry, work and worry. But how wonderful the old life seemed now! Parting with it was so unthinkable it made her scream.[4]

How do we find value in our own days of "work and worry, work and worry"? It's easy to equate ordinary days as unimportant and boring—the same routine, the same commute, the same traffic, the same work, the same problems, the same exhaustion, the same old everything. However, thinking of our everyday world as dull or insignificant is to walk through life with blinders on. The Lord Jesus commanded us to "look up" as a habit of life—to open our eyes, to be alert—and not just to His creation that surrounds us, but also to Himself and His work in us and for us. To help us look and learn, Jesus pointed out common things for our common days in the Sermon on the Mount. I imagine that from the hillside, He could literally point to these things and say, "Look at the flowers! Look at the birds!"

Consider the lilies of the field, how they grow: they neither toil nor spin, yet I tell you, even Solomon in all his glory was not arrayed like one of these.

Matthew 6:28–29

Consider the lilies—and when you do, don't think of the extra-large Easter lilies from the florist. Instead think wildflowers. Think trillium that paints the forest floor in the springtime. Or think rhododendron that bedecks a high mountain stream with pink and purple and sparks of orange, and when the wind stirs, the branches cast their crowns into the bright waters. Consider the flowers that God planted.

The flowers remind us of their Creator—and ours. They remind us that the Great Gardener purposed to give life, color, fragrance, and beauty even to wildflowers that may never be seen in their brief existence. If our God does that for flowers, He will surely be with His people, giving them His life and filling their days with the fragrance and beauty of His presence.

And just as we are to look at the flowers to grow our gratitude for God's attentive care in the day-to-day, Jesus also told us to look to the birds:

Look at the birds of the air: they neither sow nor reap nor gather into barns, and yet your heavenly Father feeds them. Are you not of more value than they?

Matthew 6:26

Are not two sparrows sold for a penny? And not one of them will fall to the ground apart from your Father. But even the hairs of your head are all numbered. Fear not, therefore; you are of more value than many sparrows.

Matthew 10:29–31

I love the story that Georgi Vins tells of when he kept company with the sparrows. Vins was a courageous Russian pastor during the Soviet era, and spent eight years in the gulags because of his Gospel work. When I met Vins late in his life, it would be the first and last time, but it was an enormously influential meeting. I was at a crossroads in my life, and Vins opened a way for me to serve Christ in Russia, Ukraine, and central Asia. It was a small opening at the time, but God would prosper it to this day.

Vins wrote of his experiences during his years in prison, and on one occasion, he wrote about what the sparrows had taught him.

Few creatures can endure the harsh climate of Siberia's far north, where the winter temperature often drops as low as -74°F. By then, the birds have long since flown south to their winter feeding grounds in the Philippines and Japan. Only the hardy ravens and magpies remain behind. And the ever-present sparrows.

During the coldest times the sparrows would cling to the sides of the barracks with their tiny claws, pressing their little bodies against the walls. There they stayed for hours. If I was very quiet, I could get close enough to see that their little eyes were closed as they rested. It was so pleasant for them. How fragile they seemed, how incongruous with the severity of our surroundings.

One day I took them some breadcrumbs. Carefully I shook the crumbs out of my pockets onto the snowy ground. Before long I was surrounded by a whole flock of sparrows and the crumbs disappeared in moments. The little birds eyed me expectantly, waiting for more. I showed them my empty hands: "I have nothing else. Tomorrow I'll try to bring you more."

After a while, the sparrows recognized me. Every time I went outside, they'd leave their precarious shelters and gather around me, waiting for their bread. There were more than I could count.

Gazing at the tiny birds, joy filled my heart as I remembered the words of the Lord Jesus Christ: "Are not two sparrows sold for a farthing? And one of them shall not fall on the ground without your Father. But the very hairs of your head are all numbered. Fear ye not therefore, ye are of more value than many sparrows" (Matthew 10:29–31).

Dear little birds, if you haven't been forgotten by God, then neither have I! And so it was during my years in bonds that I saw most clearly God's protection and His faithfulness to me and to His Word. What a privilege it is to belong to Him![5]

Similarly, when David was on the run for his life, he wrote, "The eyes of the LORD are toward the righteous and his ears toward their cry" (Psalm 34:15). Our God hears the cries of His people. Whether in the weary, dangerous years David spent waiting for God's promises to be fulfilled or in the utter obscurity of an unjust imprisonment of a pastor in Siberia, our God hears the cries of His sons and daughters. The same is true in our routine rhythms and sorrows. Our days may be too hard and our nights too long to face alone, but because of the abounding grace of Jesus, we are stronger than we know and part of something bigger than we can see.

I was reminded of this recently by a friend who shared with me an entry from her journal. Simona is a young wife and mother who wrote from inside the walls of her everyday world, where she and her husband are growing in grace and endurance and finding new boundaries of Christ's Kingdom.

Maybe we're actually doing something remarkable. Something big. Maybe what's seemed so ordinary, so slight and sometimes defeating a thing, has actually been monumental. We've made a person, kept her alive somehow, remained committed to one another and to our church through thick and much thin this year. We've talked for hours about things we wished we'd never have to think about. We've made decisions we'd never dreamed would ever exist. We've set our alarms after late nights of work and dragged ourselves out of bed to read our Bibles and pray while the dark remained and the rain came down outside for endless hours. We've had date nights in and cleaned the floors too infrequently and done five times as much laundry as we ever did before the small child.

We've stayed awake to the battle.

Each day begins where the last left off, but also seems somehow like Groundhog Day. Like we're right back where we started and the perseverance of yesterday and the day before and the day before that were all for nothing and the battle lines will remain the same for every new day.

Perhaps there is something true in that—perhaps holding the line is where the heat of the battle is at. There are times to advance and move forward, but all that means nothing if the line does not hold.

So, as we wake up each day and meet with the King and hear His words and plod through our days seeking to do justly, to love mercy, and to walk humbly with our God, our homes look more and more like outposts of that King, evidences that justice will be done, the wicked will be judged, and the righteous will be vindicated one day. Wrong will not win out in the end, but every day we have to cling to the truth anew. As we become wearied in trying to understand everything swirling around us, we must walk into the sanctuary of God to discern the end of it all. The end that makes sense of it all (Psalm 73).

And our hunger for great patience, greater peace, and more presence of God in our days as we clock into work and roll up our sleeves for another sink full of dishes, send an encouraging text to a struggling friend, and speak gently to a headstrong child—this is where the Kingdom comes. If not here, then nowhere.[6]

When the praises of God's people rise from our small but significant lives, then every day is the Lord's day. So, just as Simona is declaring from her Kingdom outpost, we pray, too,

*Lord, on this day*
  *In this appointed place*
  *Let Your Kingdom come*
  *Let Your will be done.*

# ONE DAY TO LIVE

I don't think we are in any danger, and if we are, we
might as well die suddenly in God's work as by some
long-drawn-out illness at home.[1]

—Dr. Eleanor Chesnut, in a letter written from China,
where she was martyred in 1905

*Tempus fugit*, the Latin phrase for "time flies," is a warning inscribed on the face of sundials, old clocks, and even
tombstones. It's easy to see how we get the word "fugitive" from
"fugit." Like a thief on the run, tireless time always stays just
beyond our reach. *Tempus fugit* is another way of saying "Life
is short." Life at its longest is short, but life at its shortest—
death in youth—simply takes your breath away with its speed
and indifference.

Rarely have I read a more gripping account of the truism
"life is short" than the one that Lt. Gen. John Kelly gave. Kelly,
a commander of U.S. forces in Iraq, was recommending two
Marines for posthumous decorations for valor for saving the
lives of fifty Marines and one hundred Iraqi police. Jonathan
Yale, age twenty-one, and Jordan Haerter, age nineteen, had
just taken up their posts to guard the barracks where the Marines and Iraqi security forces were asleep. Yale and Haerter

came from different units and had not met each other before standing guard at the checkpoint. A security camera recovered from the rubble captured the moment a suicide bomber and his explosives-packed truck came barreling toward the barracks—and the two Marines. General Kelly wrote:

> You can watch the last six seconds of their young lives. Putting myself in their heads I supposed it took about a second for the two Marines to separately come to the same conclusion about what was going on once the truck came into their view at the far end of the alley. Exactly no time to talk it over. . . .
>
> It took maybe another two seconds for them to present their weapons, take aim, and open up. By this time the truck was half-way through the barriers and gaining speed the whole time. . . .
>
> For about two seconds more, the recording shows the Marines' weapons firing nonstop, the truck's windshield exploding into shards of glass as their rounds take it apart and tore in to the body of the [driver] . . . who is trying to get past them to kill their brothers—American and Iraqi—bedded down in the barracks. . . .
>
> The recording shows the truck careening to a stop immediately in front of the two Marines. In all of the instantaneous violence Yale and Haerter never hesitated. By all reports and by the recording, they never stepped back. They never even started to step aside. They never even shifted their weight. With their feet spread shoulder width apart, they leaned into the danger, firing as fast as they could work their weapons. They had only one second left to live.
>
> The truck explodes. The camera goes blank. Two young men go to their God. Six seconds. Not enough time to think about their families, their country, their flag, or about their lives or their deaths, but more than enough time for two very brave young men to do their duty—into eternity.[2]

Few of us will ever find ourselves in the dangerous context in which Yale and Haerter lived and died. When *we* think of the swiftness of life, we typically think of living out our years and gradually finding (as the wrinkles and birthday candles add up) that we are caught in the same intractable predicament we heard from all the old-timers we knew growing up—that the years get shorter as we get older. We know in the end that death will come, yet we think there will be time to prepare, time to plan. Poets have often fleshed out our imagination on this point like the Appalachian ballad "O Death," where the unwelcome visitor with icy fingers is asked to reschedule for a year out. And George MacDonald wrote of looking out his window with a fright when "Yestereve, Death came, and knocked at my thin door."[3] But death—whether it comes in a fiery explosion or at the end of years of suffering—is never so polite as to knock first.

If life is short, sometimes suddenly so, then how do we respond to the inescapable? In view of the brevity and fragility of life, the fear of losing what little we have can paralyze us. Fear can become the daily bread of our existence, emptying our days of joy and any sense of adventure. All of this is given in exchange for the illusion of security. In the Age of COVID (or whatever the next threat might be), C. S. Lewis has a commonsense answer to "How then shall we live?" He was writing in 1948 when fear of an all-out nuclear war was fresh—and such peril still remains, along with a nest of other vipers that have hatched out since then—but Lewis's answer is just as relevant in the face of any number of fears that can paralyze us:

> Do not let us begin by exaggerating the novelty of our situation. Believe me, dear sir or madam, you and all whom you love were already sentenced to death before the atomic bomb was invented: and quite a high percentage of us were going to die in unpleasant ways. . . .
>
> The first action to be taken is to pull ourselves together. If we are all going to be destroyed by an atomic bomb, let that bomb when it comes find us doing sensible and human

things—praying, working, teaching, reading, listening to music, bathing the children, playing tennis, chatting to our friends over a pint and a game of darts—not huddled together like frightened sheep and thinking about bombs. They may break our bodies (a microbe can do that) but they need not dominate our minds.[4]

How do we make the most of our short lives? How do we maximize our days—these twenty-four-hour-long bits of vapor life? A fear-driven, risk-averse, comfort-zone life won't lengthen our days, and neither does a full calendar represent a full life. Some people just get more out of their twenty-four-hour days—and it's not because they never sleep. John Piper—pastor, poet, seminary founder, Christian apologist, and author of more than seventy books—would be in that "overachiever" class. In an interview about how he is able to get so much accomplished, one of his answers captured the heart of the matter:

Give ten percent of your focus in life to avoiding obstacles to productivity and ninety percent of your focus to fastening onto great goals and pursuing them with all your might. Very few people become productive by avoiding obstacles to productivity. It is not a good focus. That is not where energy comes from. It is not where vision comes from. People write books about that and make a lot of money, but that is not where anybody gets anything worthwhile done. Getting things done that count comes from great, glorious, wonderful future possibilities that take you captive and draw your pursuit with all your might. And then all that other stuff about getting obstacles out of your way, that is the ten percent of broom-work that you have to do.[5]

Pursuing "great future possibilities" against the swiftly passing backdrop of our days reminds me of a photograph I keep on my study wall because it reminds me of how dreams come true—and it's not by wishing. The photograph is of the Wright brothers' first flight. It is December 17, 1903. The flyer has just cleared the ground; Orville is at the controls, lying flat on the lower wing, and Wilbur is running alongside. The barrenness of the sand flats and dunes of Kitty Hawk stretch before them.

I bought the picture when I explored Kitty Hawk on the Outer Banks of North Carolina a few years ago. It was an unforgettable day as I walked over the vast field where men and moments of consequence passed. Here's my journal entry from that day in 2015.

Climbed to the top of Big Kill Devil Hill. From there, the ocean was in view and seagulls wheeled above and seemed to laugh at the monuments to a 12-second flight! Grass, walking paths, and a magnificent granite monument now adorn it—but when Orville and Wilbur were here, this was just a huge sand dune 100 feet high. They came to Kitty Hawk, in fact, because there was wind, sand (for softer landings), and privacy—all in abundance. The problem of flight would not be solved with equations—it

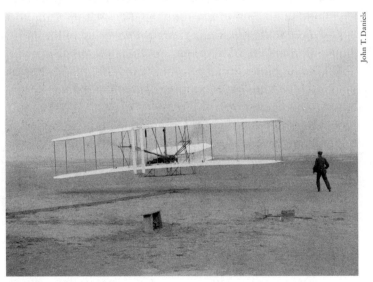

John T. Daniels

First flight

would be solved in the air. And so, in the three years before the first powered flight, here on these sand dunes, the Wright Brothers learned the ways of the wind, making over 1,000 flights in gliders.

Much has been written about the Wright Brothers' modest lives, their enormous capacity for work, and their genius—not the "Eureka!" type genius, but a steady sort of persistent problem-solving genius as they ventured further and further into the conquest of the air. Even failures were a useful—although at times painful—path to the next answer, the next breakthrough. But what interests me most is why they took the risks that they did—risks, which were real and constant, ranging from bruised ribs to sudden death. Wilbur and Orville were not daredevils, but they were daring. So, what drove them? Fame and fortune—two of the biggest reasons for taking risks—certainly weren't it. They would eventually achieve both, but that was after-the-fact. They spent their own money to pay for their venture, money drawn from the slim profits of their bicycle business in Dayton, Ohio. And they worked in obscurity. When they succeeded at Kitty Hawk, their hometown newspaper didn't even bother to print the story initially.[6] While the *Dayton Daily Journal*'s decision could be dismissed as just a small-town paper with small-town interests, even the *Scientific American* regarded the story as a hoax.[7] How could these unconnected nobodies (whose formal education went only through high school) achieve what the best minds money could buy had not?

The Wright Brothers started with a clear, simple belief about something that was actually quite unclear and complex—they believed that powered flight was possible. They didn't risk everything in order to have their names written in books or inscribed in marble. They risked everything in order to fly. There was no Plan B.

I have a friend who was also captivated by a "great future possibility"—that of spreading the fame of the Lord Jesus by putting the Bible into a language that had yet to be written for a people who had yet to hear the Good News. In the borderlands of Vietnam, Cambodia, and Laos, J.D. Crowley and his family did just that for the Tampuan people. This people, who were preliterate animists twenty-five years ago, now have thriving churches, the Tampuan Bible, a Tampuan hymnal, and a Tampuan Bible school. J.D.'s pioneer Gospel work has been done in quiet obscurity. There will be no big granite monuments to his achievements, but there will be Tampuan voices in the Kingdom choir that the apostle John saw and heard:

> And they sang a new song, saying,
> "Worthy are you to take the scroll
> and to open its seals,
> for you were slain, and by your blood you ransomed
> people for God
> from every tribe and language and people and
> nation."
>
> Revelation 5:9

J.D. has been a longtime friend, example, and encourager to me, but since his stroke and my cancer diagnosis, our times together have felt more like the camaraderie of two soldiers bloodied but still advancing. The last time J.D. wrote to me, he captured the spirit of where we are in our journey now. He closed his letter with "I love you, dear brother. Let's go into the night with defiant joy."

J.D. works in an oral culture, where storytelling is a central means of teaching. Perhaps this is why he is so gifted in explaining the parables of Jesus. His writing about one a few years ago has helped me

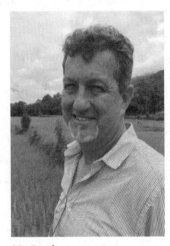

J.D. Crowley

pursue "great future possibilities" with my dwindling store of days.

I have less than one day to live. It helps me divide my life into just three stages, three "days," each one around 25 years long. The first got me past college and into marriage. The second began my adult life and took me to middle age. The sun's already rising on my third and final day that will take me to my dotage. How many days do you have left? If you're in college, the sun's already setting on your first day, and you have just two left. If you think the first day went by fast, you don't know what fast is.

The Bible piles metaphor on top of simile on top of word picture to convince you that your life is short. You're a fading flower. A mist. Grass. Dew. A shadow. Chaff. Smoke. From Job to James, God says that you will live a very, very short life followed by a very, very long eternity (Job 14:1–2; Psalm 39:4–5; 90:5–6; 103:15; James 4:14).

In light of this, I'm completely taken by Christ's story in Luke 16:1–9 about a CEO who heard that one of his managers was crooked. He called him in and fired him on the spot. Well, not quite on the spot. He gave him a little time to get his accounts in order and turned in—maybe a day, maybe two. Hmmm. Sound familiar?

What would he do with his last day? He had a plan, a shrewd plan that would impact his future. With the last bit of authority he had left, he called in everyone who owed his boss money and, to their delight, gave them huge discounts on what they owed! The boss knew he'd been beaten, but what could he do? Managers have authority to do things like that, even managers on the last day of their job. (By the way, we don't have to explain away this guy's sin; Jesus called him "dishonest" in 16:8. The point of the parable is shrewdness, not honesty.)

It sure makes it easy on the Bible student when Jesus interprets His own parable: "For the sons of this world are more shrewd in dealing with their own generation than the sons of light" (16:8). This is not a compliment to "sons of light." He's

saying we Christians are often stupid—we don't live consistently with the reality that we have just one or two "days" left
on this planet and eternity stretching out before us. The world
often lives more consistently with its values than we do. This
manager leveraged every last ounce of his rapidly-fading authority to secure great advantage for his future. He was shrewd.
How about us? Jesus implies that we're more like a manager
who spends his last day redecorating the office that he will
soon vacate.

Christ follows up His interpretation for the parable with
an application: "And I tell you, make friends for yourselves by
means of unrighteous wealth, so that when it fails they may receive you into the eternal dwellings" (16:9). Unrighteous wealth?
He's talking about your money and possessions. Eternal dwellings? He's talking about heaven! Who's going to receive you into
heaven? All those people who became your friends, and then
your brothers and sisters, because of the shrewd way you took
your tiny bit of worldly wealth and your rapidly-fading time
and leveraged them for eternal results.

It's all about Gospel leveraging. You and I don't have much.
We're not so gifted. We don't have much money. Our time's
almost gone. But that's what leveraging is all about. The Gospel
has the power to compound interest for eternity, so that even a
very small investment will yield unbelievable returns. The Lord
Jesus is telling you to take your worldly wealth and fleeting time
and put them to Gospel use. The people you impact will line the
streets to greet you when you come home to heaven. Leverage
your life for God's eternal glory and your eternal joy.[8]

As the sun of my days draws down, I still have more Gospel
leveraging ahead. I still have Kingdom dreams that cross new
borders and sound with the voices of "every tribe and language." These dreams demand risk and resoluteness. "Lord
Jesus, may the risks taken, the sacrifice of my strength and
days, display your worth alone. Keep me restless for more of
your glory until I see your face."

# STUMBLING INTO THE FUTURE

The unexpectedness of life, waiting round every corner,
catches even wise women unawares. To avoid corners
altogether is, after all, to refuse to live.[1]

—Freya Stark, *The Journey's Echo*

In the readers' guide I related a John Singer Sargent story of how the painter seized the moment given to him at the foot of the White House stairs to capture on canvas the dynamism of America's youngest president. But late in his life, Sargent captured another moment—one of even greater power and poignancy. Far from the splendor of mansions and glittering personalities, Sargent volunteered at age sixty-two to go to the Western Front in World War I to a shattered world of shattered men. His task was daunting—to capture an image that would be the centerpiece of a Hall of Remembrance to honor the sacrifice of the soldiers in the Great War.

The subject matter and the size of the work had to be epic, but what's *epic* when mired in such misery? Sargent spent weeks wandering up and down the line, waiting and wondering how he could ever capture something of the horror and the valor that swirled about him. One afternoon a British regiment was devastated in a sudden mustard gas attack. Hundreds of soldiers were lying on the ground, wounded and blinded by the gas. Orderlies helped those who could walk to an aid station—lining them up for the blind march. Sargent walked out on the scene as the sun, low in the west, washed the tragic, stumbling troop in golden light. He made quick sketches of what would become one of the most famous paintings of the war—a work simply titled "Gassed."

The composition of this painting has rightly been compared to a Greek frieze, but as I walked along the twenty-foot-long canvas in the Imperial War Museum in London, I noticed details that added sounds other than the murmurs of pain and the clumsy tramping of boots. In the distance, there are shouts of soldiers playing a pick-up game of football, and in the sky is the buzz of a dogfight, as pilots maneuvered to get in the last kill before the end of day. But ever at the forefront is Sargent's keen eye for portraying blindness—the blindness of the soldiers, the blindness of the war.

But there is something else. The painting also is an illustration of our own blindness of the future. The Scriptures tell us plainly, "You do not know what tomorrow will bring" (James 4:14). This is as true in our day-by-day lives as it is in the sudden, consequential moments of seemingly insignificant days

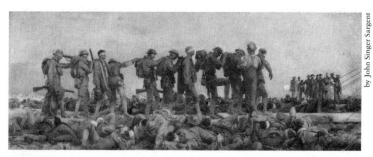

by John Singer Sargent

"Gassed"

that change the world. And we never see them coming. That was certainly the case of the day that triggered the war that Sargent documented: June 28, 1914.

I've scoured that day's Sunday edition of the *New York Times*. Were the storms of war gathering? Were diplomats being dispatched and armies mobilized? No, not yet. Macy's department store had men's summer suits on sale for $6.95, which shoppers could top off with cool straw boaters for a low price of $1.59. These ads were a reminder that vacation was just around the corner. Elsewhere in the paper, headlines told how the tough fists of boxing champ Jack Johnson had put yet another challenger on the canvas and that the Brooklyn Dodgers had made easy work of the Philadelphia Phillies in the previous day's double-header. Ironically, the newspaper's political cartoon that day was celebrating a number of successful peace initiatives by depicting a rusty, scabbarded sword. It was a comforting cartoon for that balmy summer morning in America.

Halfway around the world, however, a distant disturbance on that sleepy Sunday was destined to shake the world with an event in Sarajevo, an obscure little city on the fringe of central Europe. That day in the Austrian provincial capital promised to be gala. The Archduke Franz Ferdinand, heir to the throne of the Austro-Hungarian empire, and his wife, Sophie, were coming for a visit. The royal couple had cause for celebration, since that day was their fourteenth wedding anniversary. Beneath the flags and bunting, however, a dark scene was quietly shaping.

Seven Serbian members of the terrorist group Black Hand, who were plotting murder against the Austrians in the name of Serbian nationalism, had positioned themselves along the parade route, awaiting the archduke's motorcade. After narrowly escaping one assassin's bomb, the chauffeur took a wrong turn onto a side street, stopping the car within five feet of another of the Serbian assassins, Gavrilo Princip, who raised his small pistol and fired two quick shots. Franz Ferdinand was shot in the neck and Sophie in the abdomen. As the blood ran from her husband's mouth, Sophie cried her last frantic words, "For heaven's sake, what's happened to you?" Then, slumping over his wife's body, the dying archduke rasped his answer repeatedly, "Es ist nichts. Es ist nichts"—"It is nothing. It is nothing." The world would never be the same.

Ironically, what the archduke said was "nothing" sparked a blaze that engulfed the world. The ominous results that would come from Princip's pistol were not readily apparent, however, either in Europe or in faraway America. In the weeks to follow, the European powers, caught in a web of treaties and intrigues, were swept into war. The German emperor famously promised his parading sea of soldiers headed to the Western Front, "You will be home before the leaves have fallen from the trees." But tens of thousands of them fell before the leaves did, as the trenches of France and Flanders became mass graves for great armies. Four more summers would come and go before the bitter harvest of war was finally gathered. The body count coldly quantified the death of a generation: twenty million military and civilian deaths, along with millions more crippled for life. None of this, of course, could be seen at the onset. Like John Singer Sargent's painting of soldiers blinded by poison gas, the world stumbled into the future.

It was to be the "war to end war," but that sort of comforting rhetoric was false even before the paint dried on Sargent's blind soldiers. During the war in Bosnia in the 1990s, I was in Sarajevo when the city was still under siege by the Serbs. While there, I tracked down the spot where Princip had triggered a war. When I found the place, the street was pitted from mortar explosions, and shattered glass crunched beneath my feet. Apparently the "war to end all war" did not succeed. In addition, many of the hard realities of our world today were utterly unknown in 1914. Hitler, Stalin, Mao—the century's coming mass murderers—were just stumbling young men who had not yet figured out what they wanted to do with their lives. But there's another story of a young man stumbling into his future. Everything and everyone in this story are utterly unremarkable—except for one utterly remarkable fact: God was at work, as He always is. The future is not dark to Him. As the psalmist declares, "Even the darkness is not dark to you; the night is bright as the day, for darkness is as light with you" (Psalm 139:12). God goes before us, never stumbles, and accomplishes everything He purposes to do.

And so, on Sunday, January 6, 1850, in a little town in eastern England, a fifteen-year-old boy dutifully set out for his church, but he wasn't happy about it. Despite all the sermons he had heard and books he had read, he had no peace and no clear understanding of the Gospel. Added to that, a snowstorm struck that morning. As he leaned into the blinding wind and deepening drifts, he found his usual path impossible, so he detoured to a small church nearby. I'll let Charles Spurgeon tell you what happened next:

> I sometimes think I might have been in darkness and despair until now had it not been for the goodness of God in sending a snowstorm, one Sunday morning, while I was going to a certain place of worship. When I could go no further, I turned down a side street, and came to a little Primitive Methodist Chapel. In that chapel there may have been a dozen or fifteen people. . . . The minister did not come that morning; he was snowed up, I suppose. At last, a very thin-looking man, a shoemaker, a tailor, or something of that sort, went up into the pulpit to preach. . . . He was obliged to stick to his text, for the simple reason that he had little else to say. The text was—"Look unto Me, and be ye saved, all the ends of the earth."
>
> He did not even pronounce the words rightly, but that did not matter. There was, I thought, a glimpse of hope for me in the text. The preacher began thus: "My dear friends, this is a very

simple text indeed. It says, 'Look.' Now lookin' don't take a deal of pains. It ain't liftin' your foot or your finger; it is just 'Look.' Well, a man needn't go to College to learn to look. You may be the biggest fool, and yet you can look. A man needn't be worth a thousand a year to be able to look. Anyone can look; even a child can look. But then the text says, 'Look unto Me.' Ay, said he, in broad Essex, "many on ye are lookin' to yourselves, but it's no use lookin' there. You'll never find any comfort in yourselves." . . .

Then the good man followed up his text in this way: "Look unto Me: I am sweatin' great drops of blood. Look unto Me; I am hangin' on the cross. Look unto Me; I am dead and buried.

Look unto Me; I rise again. Look unto Me; I ascend to Heaven; look unto Me; I am sittin' at the Father's right hand. O poor sinner, look unto Me! Look to Me!"

When he had got about that length, and managed to spin out ten minutes or so, he was at the length of his tether. Then he looked at me under the gallery, and I daresay, with so few present, he knew me to be a stranger. Just fixing his eyes on me, as if he knew all my heart, he said, "Young man, you look very miserable." Well, I did, but I had not been accustomed to have remarks made from the pulpit on my personal appearance before. However, it was a good blow, struck right home. He continued, "and you always will be miserable—miserable in life, and miserable in death—if you don't obey my text; but if you obey now, this moment, you will be saved." Then, lifting up his hands, he shouted, as only a Primitive Methodist could do, "Young man, look to Jesus Christ. Look! Look! Look! You have nothin' to do but to look and live." . . .

There and then the cloud was gone, the darkness had rolled away, and that moment I saw the sun; and I could have risen that instant, and sung with the most enthusiastic of them, of the precious blood of Christ, and the simple faith which looks alone to Him.[2]

The day Charles Spurgeon was converted would make an everlasting difference—one greater than wars and politics. For there is nothing more powerful or permanent than a life transformed and driven by the Gospel. "And those who are wise shall shine like the brightness of the sky above; and those who turn many to righteousness, like the stars forever and ever" (Daniel 12:3).

It is significant that God would use an insignificant day, an insignificant messenger humble and unknown, and an insignificant teenager to accomplish His saving work. God was writing the story of that day—and He was not stumbling. He was leading. He is in charge of snowstorms and the steps of a troubled teenager. God always knows the way ahead because, as Samuel Zwemer wrote, "He is . . . 'the Great Opener.' He opens the lips of the dumb to song, the eyes of the blind to sight, and the prison house to the captive. He opens the doors of utterance and entrance for the Gospel. He opens graves and gates, the windows of heaven and the bars of death. He holds all the keys of every situation."[3] As in all the days recorded in this book—and all the unknown ones ahead—the Shepherd with scars in His hands takes the lead so that we need not stumble.

On those days when our strength fails, when our plans lie in pieces, when tears cloud the hope and glory beyond us, then this Good Shepherd lifts us up for a better view, and He carries us on.

# TIME IN A RECTANGLE

Most of what happens to us goes unremembered. The events of our lives are like photographic negatives. The few that make it into the developing solution and become photographs are what we call our memories.[1]

—Janet Malcolm in *Still Pictures*

Back there at the beginning, as I see now, my life was all time and almost no memory. . . . And now, nearing the end, I see that my life is almost entirely memory and very little time.[2]

—Jayber Crow, in Wendell Berry's *Jayber Crow*

My neighbor Wick McKain is a good storyteller—and at ninety-seven, his stories span much of the past century. He still lives in the house that he and his wife built after he came back from the war. There is a fence between our two properties, but I added a gate to it. If fences make good neighbors, then I figure a gate makes an even better neighbor. Wick is still quite independent, but I check in on him as often as I can. It's easy for us to while away an hour talking—catching up on family news, comparing notes on the butterflies we've seen, or planning our next outing to Waffle House.

But my favorite conversations with Wick are in the past tense. Wick can talk about the Great Depression from experience—not just from history books. He remembers Franklin Roosevelt's fireside chats on his family's prized radio, but mostly he remembers life in the Southern mill village where he grew up and how people worked together to survive—even plowing up the baseball field to plant black-eyed peas so there would be enough for everyone to eat.

Wick graduated from high school in 1943, and within a week he was off to war. He volunteered for the Navy, where he served as a turret gunner on a bomber in the war against Germany. Not long ago, he brought out a picture of him as a young Navy airman, and I saw that the nearly eighty years that separated the photo from the person in front of me had not erased his smile! The essayist Lance Morrow wrote that a photograph "imprisons [time] in rectangles." It freezes a moment but can never tell the whole story.[3] I know that beyond that handsome sailor's wartime portrait were tears as well as smiles, because Wick's

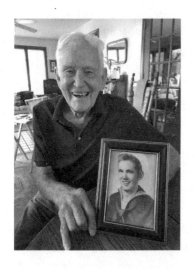

days as a turret gunner—dodging and dispensing death—live on in vivid memories and flashbacks of haunting faces that rise from the fog of a long-ago battle.

We were having supper at Waffle House one evening recently when the kaleidoscope of conversation turned to the day the war ended. War in Europe was over, but the final fight to defeat Japan lay ahead, and that's where Wick was headed. He had survived two years of combat, but would his luck hold out? It was a depressing prospect, but duty called. Wick was headed toward his rendezvous with the Pacific war when news broke that Japan had surrendered. Suddenly, he knew he had survived the war and was going home! Wick recalled every detail of Victory Day, this day of deliverance for him and millions of others. Like the legendary kiss in Eisenstaedt's famous photograph, spontaneous celebrations broke out in the streets with raucous joy, and Wick was caught up in one of them. He looked at me across the table, his eyes glistening with all that he was seeing, and he said, "Where were you that day?" Taken back by the question and his genuine eagerness to know, I said, "Wick, I wasn't born yet."

Suddenly, he came back from that shining memory to the corner booth where we were sitting at Waffle House. Wick was a little embarrassed, but I thought it was a beautiful, unconscious act of friendship, for this was a memory so big, alive, and happy that he thought I must have been in it somehow.

Frederick Buechner captures this powerful conjuring force of memory that each of us carries inside:

> Every person we have ever known, every place we have ever seen, everything that has ever happened to us—it all lives and breathes deep in us somewhere whether we like it or not, and sometimes it doesn't take much to bring it back to the surface in bits and pieces. A scrap of some song that was popular years ago. A book we read as a child. A stretch of road we used to travel. An old photograph, an old letter. There is no telling what trivial thing may do it, and then suddenly there it all is . . . Times too beautiful to tell or too terrible. Memories come at us helter-skelter and unbidden, sometimes so thick and fast that they are more than we can handle in their poignancy, sometimes so sparsely that we all but cry out to remember more.[4]

Memory, like photographs, captures our past in its own kind of rectangle—setting the bounds of where we've come from and what has become of us. Danville, Virginia, is a river town where the muddy Dan meanders past old cotton mills and redbrick warehouses the color of the southern clay they came from. It wends on beneath the bridges and train trestles I know so well and past a great green hill where my mama and my daddy are buried.

My earliest memories are bound up in a one-square-mile patch along that river. My house, my school, my church, and the woods where I played were all there, along with a creek called Dead Man's Creek, which was at the bottom of Dead Man's Cliff. After I grew up and saw more of the world and its ways, I learned—to my deep disappointment—that every other kid who found a creek in the woods also named it "Dead Man's Creek." The last time I ventured back to the *original* Dead Man's Creek, it was flowing through concrete culverts with a subdivision all around it. These people have no idea what rich boyhood history their shiny cookie-cutter houses now sit astride, nor what ghosts stir along that storied ridge formerly known as Dead Man's Cliff.

The centerpiece of my world was, of course, my house with its row of apple trees, a garden, a goldfish pond, a great catawba tree—with enough room left for backyard baseball. The house was well loved and, therefore, well lived in. Even now I can recall every inch of every room—the worn red carpet, the stacks of books, and the clutter of family photographs. I can still hear my mother's singing at the piano on Saturday nights and see my father coming home from the machine shop where he worked, his shirt stained with grease and his strong hands smelling of steel.

Despite my love for this place and the bit of earth it occupies, I dreamed of traveling far, far from it—and that dream came true. But I kept a house key and went back as often as I could because there was always a place waiting for me at my mama's table. I often felt like Bilbo when he returned to the Shire at the end of his battles and footsore adventures:

60

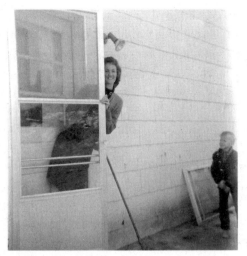

With Mama at our door, 1964

Roads go ever ever on
  Under cloud and under star,
Yet feet that wandering have gone
  Turn at last to home afar.
Eyes that fire and sword have seen
  And horror in the halls of stone
Look at last on meadows green
  And trees and hills they long have known.[5]

But those homecomings didn't last. My mother died in 2005, and my father lived on at the house until his death there in 2013. My brother and sisters and I all had our own places and lives, so the old homestead was cleaned out and sold. Afterwards, when I came back to visit family, I would not—could not—drive down the street where I grew up, much less look at the house. For nearly ten years I stayed away, but one day I was back in my hometown and thought, *Why not make peace with this place? Why not go back home?* And so, I did. I drove along the river and made the few turns that led to the old neighborhood. My truck wheels seemed to fall into familiar lines. I could have driven it with my eyes closed, but I kept them wide open to take in the place I knew so well. And suddenly, there it was. My old house.

Sometimes we do things we know will hurt. We think it will bring closure, but mostly it just hurts. It wasn't just that the trees were all cut down or my mother's flowers gone without a trace or the obvious neglect of the house. The real hurt was I knew if I knocked on the familiar door, a stranger would answer—an intruder into my house of memory. The house was there and the address the same, but I might as well have been on the wrong street in another city. The place I knew so well could now be unlocked only with memory's key. I shouldn't have been—but I was—shaken by how transient it all is. I know that we are to "fix our eyes not on what is seen, but on what is unseen, since what is seen is temporary, but what is unseen is eternal" (2 Corinthians 4:18 NIV) and that life, as James described, is "a mist that appears for a little while and then vanishes" (James 4:14 NIV). I know all that, but still the moment struck hard with loss as all the solid-seeming bits of my past were turning to mist in this passing-away world, and the losses of my mother and father were vivid again. Going back was like throwing another shovelful of dirt on their graves.

As I drove away in heaviness, the truck wheels again seemed to fall into familiar lines—and soon I found myself at the little church where I grew up. It was the middle of a weekday, so all was quiet. I tested the locked door and found it had not been pulled completely closed. I pushed it open, and it was like entering a time capsule. Other than the date on last Sunday's bulletins left in the foyer, it could have been fifty years ago. I sat on the back pew of the choir loft and took in the whole sanctuary. I remember sitting here Sunday after Sunday and hearing the Gospel preached with such clarity and power. And I remember clearly the night I believed on the Lord Jesus and how on my way home, I stood beneath a star-filled sky and knew that Christ had forgiven all my sins and felt the rush of freedom like a pardoned prisoner who suddenly finds that not only has his name been cleared, but he has been loaded with titles of honor: beloved, heir, son!

As I thought of that night, the lines of Wesley's hymn we used to sing came to mind:

> My chains fell off,
> My heart was free,
> I rose, went forth,
> And followed Thee.[6]

And I remembered the lines of a favorite hymn that echoed there many a Sunday:

> Blessed assurance, Jesus is mine!
> Oh, what a foretaste of glory divine!
> Heir of salvation, purchase of God,
> born of his Spirit, washed in his blood.
> This is my story, this is my song,
> praising my Savior all the day long.[7]

These are the memories rooted in grace that led to more lasting things. As Peter said, "According to his great mercy, he has caused us to be born again to a living hope through the resurrection of Jesus Christ from the dead, to an inheritance that is imperishable, undefiled, and unfading" (1 Peter 1:3–4). Unfading—unlike pictures, places, and the people I once held in my arms. My longings for home, held now only in the shadows of memory, will be found in their full, unfading glory not in my little house but in my Father's house. *This* is my story. *This* is my song.

# ALONG THE WAY

I shot an arrow into the air,
It fell to earth, I knew not where;
For, so swiftly it flew, the sight
Could not follow in its flight.

I breathed a song into the air,
It fell to earth, I knew not where;
For who has sight so keen and strong,
That it can follow the flight of song?

Long, long afterward, in an oak
I found the arrow, still unbroke;
And the song, from beginning to end,
I found again in the heart of a friend.[1]

—Henry Wadsworth Longfellow,
"The Arrow and the Song"

# IN THE EYE OF A STORM

I will sing of your strength; I will sing aloud of your
steadfast love in the morning. For you have been to me
a fortress and a refuge in the day of my distress.

—Psalm 59:16

We were scheduled to pass through the Pillars of Hercules
at daybreak. As a Navy cadet in 1974, I was making
my first Atlantic crossing. Seeing the Rock of Gibraltar in the
light of red dawn—and two continents at a glance—would
have been a voyager's dream come true. I had passed the night
hours caught between waking and sleeping. Too impatient for
the alarm, I dressed and went up on the deck at 4:30 to see this
glorious horizon.

But I couldn't see anything.

Heavy fog shrouded the strait. I could see only a few steps
away along the ship's deck, and so I worked my way up to the
bridge to see what I could see. The Strait of Gibraltar is a choke
point—the maritime equivalent of going from sixteen lanes to
two—and large ships can't maneuver easily in a blind fog. All
around us, unseen ships were blaring their horns, as were we.
It was like a traffic jam, only driving blind. The bridge was
aswirl as sailors peered into the murk from the port and star-
board watches; others studied the radar screen, and there was

a huddle about the helmsman. But in the midst of this tense, tight hurry sat the captain.

Richard Dewey was always the picture of an old-school Navy captain. Behind his spit-and-polish exterior was a combat-hardened commander. He exuded strength without trying, and he was the kind of warrior that men follow into battle because he leads the way. But on this fog-shrouded morning, I remember he was wearing slippers, sitting back in his chair, and sipping coffee. An officer would come to him and report. Orders were quietly given, and the lieutenant was off in a flash as the captain returned to his morning cup.

I didn't get to see two continents at a glance that morning, but I did get an unforgettable glimpse of calm command. Jesus is like that. When circumstances are out of our control (and they always are) and threats sound from the darkness, Christ our Captain is at the center of it—unshaken, unhurried, undaunted, sovereign in His control, and steadfast in His love.

Rosaria Butterfield describes her conversion as "the peace inside the eye of a hurricane."[1] It's a good description, for fierce storms have swirled about her since the day she believed on Jesus. She has been struck by their rage, but the center has held because her Captain is there and has written promises in blood that He will never leave her.

Rosaria was a tenured professor, a radical feminist, a leader in the LGBTQ community, and was herself a committed lesbian. She despised Christians for what they stood for. And of the Christians she had encountered, the feeling was mutual. That is, until she met Ken and Floy Smith. Ken was a pastor in Syracuse, New York, near the university where Rosaria taught. The Smiths did not invite Rosaria to their church, at least not for a while. They first invited her to their home for a meal and conversation. What followed was two years of meals and conversations, during which the Spirit of God gave a pastor and his wife words of Gospel wisdom as well as genuine, unhurried, disarming grace.

But the Spirit of God was working on both sides of the dinner table as Rosaria reached a crisis point in her path as she encountered the Way, the Truth, and the Life. One night, her own raging ceased as she entered the eye of the hurricane. "I prayed, and asked God if the Gospel message was for someone like me, too. I viscerally felt the living presence of God as I prayed. Jesus seemed present and alive. I knew that I was not alone in my room. I prayed that if Jesus was truly a real and risen God, that he would change my heart. And if he was real and if I was his, I prayed he would give me the strength of mind to follow him and the character to become a godly woman. I prayed for the strength of character to repent for a sin that at that time didn't feel like sin at all—it felt like life plain and simple. I prayed that if my life was actually his life, that he would take it back and make it what he wanted it to be. I asked him to take it all: my sexuality, my profession, my community, my tastes, my books, and my tomorrows."[2]

I found Rosaria still living, serving, and shining in the eye of a hurricane when I spent a day with her and her family.

**Durham, North Carolina**
**Sunday, June 7, 2020**

Out in the kitchen the sounds of coffee grinding and lovely humming were my morning greeting. Rosaria was stirring up some breakfast while her husband, Kent, was in a quiet corner working on final sermon prep. Their two teenagers, Knox and Mary, were squeezing the last bit of sleep out of the night before a flurry of chores and church. Even though I rose with the sun, Rosaria, as is her practice, was already up by five, since for her, early morning is always a time of prayer. In these earliest hours, she spends time in five psalms—praying through them, sometimes singing through them from a psalter. One of the psalms in her reading this morning was Psalm 68, and this verse stood out: "Blessed be the Lord, who daily bears us up; God is our salvation" (v. 19). Among her Bible, psalter, and prayer lists lay a book of 365 devotionals open to June 7. Words from the old Puritan Thomas Manton were underlined. "God would have us come every day to the throne of grace. Our mercies do not flow from God all at once, but some today, and others tomorrow. All together they are too heavy for us to wield and manage. Our mercies come in great numbers, but God distributes them by parcels that we are able to acknowledge them and be thankful for them."[3] A parcel of mercy—what a beautiful way to describe this day!

I was most interested to see Rosaria's prayer journal—a simple spiral-bound tablet with headings such as "Family," "Neighbors," "Nation," "Church Family," "Prisoners," "Urgent," each with a list of names she prays through every day. Highlighter and penciled updates mark the progress of her prayer-work done over these worn pages. The first page of her prayer journal—and the first to be prayed for each morning—was under the heading "Prayer for my enemies." The page was full of names.

After a generous round of scrambled eggs, bacon, and a second cup, Kent headed over to church while Rosaria and I took their dogs out for their morning walk. I walked Bella—or she walked me. Bella is a perky little Shih Tzu, and knowing I was the new kid on the block, she took charge. Rosaria walked Sully, a sweet, goofy three-legged mutt rescued from the animal shelter seven years before. Born with only one foreleg, Sully lunges as he walks, but his limitation doesn't keep him from chasing squirrels or even deer on our walk. Even though he was forever always hopelessly behind in every pursuit, Sully is indefatigable! That Rosaria took in a three-legged dog that no one else wanted seems entirely fitting.

As we made our way around the neighborhood, we passed others out for a morning jog or walking their dogs. Even though

we were several blocks from her
house, Rosaria called them all
by name—sometimes asking a
quick question about a child's
health situation or the status of
a job search. All of these passing
conversations represent deeper
stories and long-term invest-
ments in loving her neighbors.
Rosaria has a saying: "God
never gets the address wrong."
That is, our Sovereign King posi-
tions His servants to serve Him.
And that means it's neither the

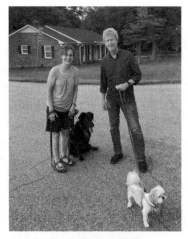

With Rosaria, Sully, and Bella

blame nor the credit of the real estate agent as to where we live.
It's no accident who lives across the street, around the corner,
or in the apartment above us. So, Rosaria and Kent's place is
their special sovereign assignment, and these winding streets
that connect Rosaria and her family with a hundred households
are the King's Highway. From here, by prayer, open hands, an
open door, an open table, and an open Bible, it's possible for
strangers to become neighbors—and neighbors become family.

After getting Sully and Bella settled back home, Rosaria,
Knox, Mary, and I headed over to church—First Reformed Presbyterian Church—where Kent pastors. Most of the churches in
the area were still closed because of the pandemic, but while
taking reasonable precautions and social distancing, the saints
here were gathering to worship. So the great oak doors of the
church were opened, and young Knox took his place at the
entrance to greet all who came. There was a good gathering
that morning—despite both coronavirus fears and the violence
and looting that had roiled the area in the wake of the protests
following George Floyd's death. Those who came weren't just
church members, but believers from other churches as well.

Rosaria called them "pilgrims" because they gathered there since their churches weren't meeting together yet.

The service was both ancient and modern. It was ancient in the simplicity of its elements (prayer, the breaking of bread, the preaching of the Word, and the unaccompanied singing of the Psalms). There were no instruments—just the instruments of voices accustomed to singing the ancient texts together. And the service was modern, as Kent applied the Word to our needs today and pointed us all to Christ, who continues to save sinners.

Kent was preaching through Mark's Gospel, and that day he was in chapter 15. Kent walked us through the violent swirl of events surrounding the crucifixion—the injustice of the mob, the cruelty of the Roman soldiers, the pitiless mocking of a man as He slowly bled to death, the shame of nakedness, the agony of thirst. I thought of the meditation written by Lancelot Andrewes long ago:

> By Thy sweat bloody and clotted!
> Thy soul in agony,
> Thy head crowned with thorns, bruised with staves,
> Thine eyes a fountain of tears,
> Thine ears full of insults,
> Thy mouth moistened with vinegar and gall,
> Thy face stained with spitting,
> Thy neck bowed down with the burden of the Cross,
> Thy back ploughed with the wheals and wounds of the
>     scourge,
> Thy pierced hands and feet,
> Thy strong cry, Eli, Eli,
> Thy heart pierced with the spear,
> The water and blood thence flowing,
> Thy body broken, Thy blood poured out -
> Lord forgive the iniquity of Thy servant
> And cover all his sin.[4]

This is the mystery and majesty of sovereign grace. Christ on the Cross—in the center of a torrent of evil against Him—became our peace. As Isaiah said, "But he was pierced for our transgressions; he was crushed for our iniquities; upon him was the chastisement that brought us peace, and with his wounds we are healed" (Isaiah 53:5). And again, Paul wrote, "But now in Christ Jesus you who once were far off have been brought near by the blood of Christ. For he himself is our peace" (Ephesians 2:13–14). Jesus is the "eye of the hurricane" that Rosaria entered the day she believed. And this is the peace that filled me with fresh joy as we sang the parting psalm "Praise the Lord" from *The Book of Psalms for Worship*:

> He who has the God of Jacob
> As his help is truly blessed.
> On the Lord his God forever
> Will his hope securely rest.[5]

A homeless man had slipped in during the service and sat in the back. At the close, Rosaria welcomed him and asked how they could help. He was hungry and thirsty, and she gave him soup and bread from the lunch they had brought to church today. She also washed and refilled his water bottle while he went into the men's room to wash his hands and wash out his sweaty T-shirt. The man was refreshed and grateful and listened as Kent shared the Gospel with him. What was striking was how comfortable they were with all of this, and their ease put this stranger at ease.

Rosaria's love for strangers (the literal meaning of our word *hospitality*[6]) is driven by the Gospel and by experience—for she, too, was once a stranger in church. In Rosaria's spiritual autobiography—her version of John Bunyan's *Grace Abounding to the Chief of Sinners*—she wrote about that first Sunday some twenty years prior when she was the stranger in church with her butch haircut and her truck in the parking lot with gay rights and abortion rights bumper stickers proudly on display. "That morning—February 14, 1999—I emerged from the bed of my lesbian lover and an hour later was sitting in a pew at the Syracuse Reformed Presbyterian Church. I share this detail with you not to be lurid but merely to make the point that you never know the terrain that someone else has walked to come worship the Lord."[7] Her sympathy for strangers, for seekers and outsiders, is strong because she has sat where they sit.

This afternoon some of the folks at church came to the Butterfields' home, while others from the neighborhood drifted in. Many well-worn paths lead to this house, and I expected most would stay for dinner. And from the aroma of the simmering pot roast, I was all in, too! Their open door and places at the table are the radically ordinary hospitality that adorns Rosaria and Kent's Gospel witness.

There's a passage in one of Rosaria's books about two ways Christians often respond to a post-Christian culture that meets them with contempt at every turn. These responses are driven by fear and anger, which are two sides of the same fallen coin:

> One option is to build the walls higher, declare more vociferously that our homes are our castles, and, since the world is going to hell in a handbasket, we best get inside, thank God for the moat, and draw up the bridge. Doing so practices war on this world but not the kind of spiritual warfare that drives out darkness and brings in the kindness of the gospel. . . .
>
> Our other option is to despise the blood of Christ and reinvent a Christianity that fits nicely on the "coexist" bumper sticker, avoiding the disgrace and shame of the cross for a respectable religion that bows to the idols of our day: consumerism and sexual autonomy. This manipulation strategy relies on using biblical words in anti-biblical ways. It shares with biblical Christianity the same vocabulary but not the same dictionary. This option is equally dreadful, and prevalent.[8]

But Rosaria and Kent have chosen another way—not simply random acts of kindness but a day-in, day-out living sacrifice way that reaches people where they are with a Gospel that does not leave them as they are. Their hospitality isn't an evangelistic trap or a tidy, Instagrammable event. Their hospitality toward messed-up people—whether a meth addict or the church-going type—is the overflow of the abundant mercy they, too, needed and received. And so, I hear echoes of Jude in this place: "And have mercy on those who doubt; save others by snatching them out of the fire; to others show mercy with fear, hating even the garment stained by the flesh" (Jude 1:22–23).

The kitchen was lively when I entered in search of coffee. Rosaria was in the middle of the action—cooking and counseling—as half a dozen joined in to help and to listen. A big steamer of rice was going, *dal* was in the works, and the roast was calling me. Next to the kitchen is Knox and Mary's homeschool classroom, where eight chickens were being raised in a big cardboard corral. I can't remember all their names, but one was General Heather Feather-Foot (I take it she rules the roost!), and another was a golden chicken ominously named Nugget. Sully and a big orange cat named Caspian lurked at the gated threshold from time to time, so everyone was more or less on "Chicken Patrol."

I've always felt that over time, houses absorb something of the character of their owners—not just in the objects or furniture, but in deeper ways. The conversation, laughter, screams, tears, and sunshine are absorbed in the walls, stairs, and windowsills. The contentment and comfort that make a place a refuge—or the anger, abuse, and ugly secrets that make a house a hell—soak in like stain into wood. It's just a sense—like smell and taste—but I have a sense of place. And that afternoon my sense in those rooms was of peace. Here the Word had been read and rehearsed and repented over, and the songs of David had echoed and entered these walls and hearts. How many parcels of mercy (to use

Manton's words) had been unpacked here? This cheerful—and occasionally chaotic—place is a home that many who do not live here can come to and feel safe and welcome. They are drawn by the winsomeness of Christ that fills the place like the sunshine that poured through the windows on that clear afternoon.

When dinner was ready, we gathered around a long, sturdy old table—a family piece passed down to Kent through five generations. These days this table is much more than century-old mahogany and Chippendale curves. It is where the laws of love—love God with all your heart, soul, and mind, *and* love your neighbor as yourself—are embraced and served up with second helpings and good gravy.

There were more than twenty of us sharing dinner. Sixteen of us snugged around the great table, and the younger ones sat at another table in an adjoining room. There were brothers and sisters in Christ along with wanderers, outcasts, and kids from deeply dysfunctional homes, including one whose dad was in prison.

All of us were served well. After the meal and conversations wound down, the table was cleared and Bibles and psalters were passed around to those who wanted to stay. Among the psalms we sang was Psalm 80. It was Rosaria's choice in this time of global and national chaos, as well as the brokenness and sin in our churches, homes, and hearts. Rosaria simply said, "This is where we are," and then she led us in "Hear, O Hear Us" from *The Book of Psalms for Worship*:

> Hear, O hear us, Isr'el's Shepherd,
> Who drives forth Joseph like a flock.
> From the cherubim, O shine forth;
> Rise in valor that we be saved.
> So arise in sight of Ephraim,
> And Manasseh and Benjamin.
> God, we pray, O turn us, bring us back;
> Shine Your face on us, we'll be saved.

O how long, Lord God of Armies
Burns Your wrath at Your people's prayer?
With the bread of tears You feed them,
And full measure of tears they drink.
Strife You make us to our neighbors,
And our foes laugh at us in scorn.
God of Armies, turn us, bring us back;
Shine Your face on us, we'll be saved.[9]

Rosaria's voice has a lilting loveliness with a childlike intimacy about it. The psalm's lyrics finished by pointing us to Christ, the Son of Man, our only hope.

Lay Your hand on him You favored,
Son of man that you raised in strength.
Then from You we will not wander;
Make us live; we will call Your name.
O Lord God of Armies, turn us back;
Shine Your face on us, we'll be saved![10]

Then Rosaria quietly said again—to us, to herself, and to Jesus—"This is where we are."

Afterwards, Rosaria and I took another walk with Sully and Bella. The streets were quiet and the shadows lengthening. It was a good time to talk. One of the things that had been on my mind all day to ask her about was the first and full page of her prayer list that I saw under the heading "Prayer for my enemies." It is not a blacklist of those who crossed her the wrong way, but rather a prayer list for those who have made themselves the enemy of Christ and made her family the target of their hate. I asked what Rosaria prays for her enemies, and she said she prays for conversion, for the opportunity to do them good, and that she will be careful not to sin against them.

She went on to explain to me the background of the most recent round of attacks. A couple of weeks prior, Rosaria had written an article for Desiring God about God's sovereignty over the pandemic and about one of the million ways He had opened extraordinary Gospel advances in new opportunities she and her church family had had to reach their community. She also pointed out something else that was unprecedented:

> COVID-19 also has sharpened my theological understanding of good and evil, providence and calamity, sin and repentance, belief in Christ and grace. . . . Giving thanks to God for everything, including COVID-19, humbles us—deeply. It reminds us that God's providence is perfect and our point of view flawed. Because God is good, just, and wise, all the time and in every circumstance, then COVID-19, for the Christian, must be for our good and for God's glory.
>
> Giving thanks to God for COVID-19 also positions us to begin to see the world from his point of view. The pandemic destroys our idols of prosperity, breaks down the false confidence of all men, and makes us all feel unsafe in our own strength—and feeling unsafe is sensible. As John Calvin writes in his commentary on Hosea 1:5, "There is no reason why we should feel safe when God declares himself opposed to and angry with us."
>
> The idols that God is destroying are both national and personal. God is pointing his finger at all of our hearts. If taking away our prosperity is how God will shake us up from our national and personal sins, are we all in?
>
> Have you considered the ramifications that this June will be the first in decades without a public gay pride march? Why is this big news? First, sexual identity depends on an affirming audience who can sway others to its side, using an ideology of personal freedom and victimhood. A virtual platform draws only the faithful, denying them the oxygen that this particular fire needs. Second, without an audience, sexual identity cannot be normalized.[11]

This article unleashed a fury of filthy, violent threats against her and the church by a militant group within the LGBTQ movement. When the threats started, John Piper called to check on her and to pray with her and Kent. Piper asked Rosaria what she feared the most. She answered that she was afraid she wouldn't have conduct that's becoming of a pastor's wife. John had a good laugh over that and said, "Your conduct adorns you as a pastor's wife!"

But that was just the latest storm, for Rosaria's life and ministry have been a battle from the start. She remembers that Ken Smith, her pastor at the time of her conversion, warned her, "You know this is going to be hard, don't you? You are David and Daniel and Paul—and you will be attacked." Since Rosaria was a radical professor and advocate for the LGBTQ community, her deep ties in that world—her friends, her lesbian partner, her leadership—all made her a special target. As it was said of early Christians, Rosaria turned their world upside down when Christ made her His own.

Just as Christ loved His enemies, so Rosaria, in following her Cross-bearer, could and would love His enemies, too—even when that put her squarely in their line of fire. Not surprisingly, Rosaria's background and her ability to decode the deceit surrounding sexual identity brought out their hate. But her bold witness to the Gospel of grace that crosses every kind of barrier has also disturbed and exposed the hatred in the hearts of Christians for God's image-bearers who are lost, confused, and cut off in their homosexuality. So she gets hit from both sides. I guess that's why there are so many names on her first-to-be-prayed-for list.

Rosaria said that during times of protests or when death threats come out of the darkness, she makes a quiet place—whether backstage or on her back porch—and sings a portion of Psalm 119 from the psalter:

> O let Your loving kindnesses
> Now come to me, O Lord;
> May Your salvation also come,
> According to Your word.

Then I shall answer him who taunts,
For in Your word I trust.
Take not the true word from my mouth;
I trust Your judgments just.

Your testimonies kings will hear,
I'll speak them unashamed.
Yes, I delight in Your commands;
For they my love have claimed.[12]

We had a good walk and talk. Sully was winded but happy as he lunged along the home stretch. The light was dusky blue and spangled with the first fireflies. The day, this "parcel of mercy," had been filled with good things, and the mercy and kindness on display throughout Rosaria's days are but a glimmer of the abundant, surprising, pursuing mercy of Jesus. Rosaria's conversion was the radical claim of His sovereign love. That such a person who, like the apostle Paul, was an "insolent opponent" (1 Timothy 1:13) could today be a pastor's wife and mom, as well as an outspoken, outstanding witness to the risen Christ should be a warning to all enemies of the Cross that they are not safe in the dark. As Mr. Beaver reminded the wide-eyed Lucy about the great lion Aslan, "Safe? . . . Who said anything about safe? 'Course he isn't safe. But he's good. He's the King, I tell you."[13]

# DAY OF HOPEFUL PLANTING

> Then, said he, I am going to my Father's, and tho' with
> great difficulty I am got hither, yet now I do not repent
> me of all the trouble I have been at to arrive where I
> am. *My Sword* I give to him that shall succeed me in my
> Pilgrimage, and my *Courage* and *Skill* to him that can get
> it. My *marks* and *scars* I carry with me, to be a witness
> for me, that I have fought His battles, who now will be
> my Rewarder. When the day that he must go hence was
> come, many accompany'd him to the River-side, into
> which as he went, he said, *Death, where is thy Sting?*
> And as he went down deeper, he said, *Grave, where is
> thy Victory?* So he passed over, and all the Trumpets
> sounded for him on the other side.[1]
>
> —Mr. Valiant-for-Truth in *The Pilgrim's Progress*

Looking back, it seems the tide turned for my friend Jonathan Henning sometime in the colorless winter days of 2020. For over two years, he was in a fight for his life, parrying multiple blows as cancer spread throughout his body—bladder, bone, liver, lungs, and brain. Remarkably, throughout the previous year, he had continued to work at the auto shop where he was a mechanic, while also juggling appointments, undergoing treatments, fighting nausea, and strengthening the faith of all of us who knew him. Yet cancer's steady march of misery eventually overtook him. Those last months with Jonathan were for me something like entering the holy of holies—for it is a sacred thing to walk with a saint until they reach home. By life and death, they remind us of realities. It's not just the reality that we, too, are going to die someday—a walk through a cemetery can do that. But a saint's death reminds us of even greater realities, for we get glimpses of our risen King and the power and glory of His unending life, which He also gives to His people.

John Bunyan pictured death for the Christian as crossing a river. Yet the river meant more than death. It also meant deliverance—final, complete, promised deliverance—for a mighty welcome awaits on the farther shore, where "He will wipe away every tear from their eyes, and death shall be no more, neither shall there be mourning, nor crying, nor pain anymore, for the former things have passed away" (Revelation 21:4). Jonathan reminds me of one of the characters in *The Pilgrim's Progress*: Mr. Standfast. Unlike other heaven-bound pilgrims that Bunyan described—some of whom were swept up in a chariot or swam the stream swiftly—Mr. Standfast waded in and stood for a time and ministered to those Christians along the banks of that fearful place.[2] That is how Jonathan in his last months served his family, his friends, his neighbors, and his fellow cancer patients. If medals were awarded for battling cancer, Jonathan would have received a medal of honor for courage, hope, and lifting others who had fallen.

Yet, the way across the river is still daunting. Dying is hard because we were made to live. There are fears, pain, sobbing tears, and dark doubts in the valley of the shadow of death. But for the one who belongs to Jesus, there is also strong hope and death-defying joy—both for the one crossing the river and for those still on this side of the shore. Such sweet consolation is bound up in the resurrection.

There's a brilliant passage in one of George Herbert's poems. It's a vision that looks beyond the grave but is mindful of the tears that fall on this side of it.

> Awake sad heart, whom sorrow ever drowns;
>   Take up thine eyes, which feed on earth;
> Unfold thy forehead, gather'd into frowns:
>   Thy Saviour comes, and with Him mirth:
>     Awake, awake;
> And with a thankful heart His comforts take.
>   But thou dost still lament, and pine, and cry;
>   And feel His death, but not his victory.
>   . . . . . . . . . . . . .
>     Arise, arise;
> And with His burial-linen dry thine eyes:
>   Christ left His grave-clothes, that we might when grief
>   Draws tears, or blood, not want a handkerchief.[3]

No single day could capture the ordinary beauty in this bitter providence. Also, the severity of Jonathan's pain made only brief visits possible. Early on, he made a joke whenever I asked if I could come over for a visit. In a twist on a line from the old hymn "Come Ye Sinners," Jonathan would always reply, "If you tarry till I'm better, you will never come at all." So I did not tarry but took every opportunity to be by his side—walking together, then sitting together, then just holding his hand. Here are glimpses from seven days we shared at the river's edge.

### April 25

Jonathan had something he wanted to tell me. When I came by his house, he was out back in his garden. He shared that the latest round of chemotherapy to slow the cancer had not worked. A flurry of therapies the past several months to deal with multiple cancers had failed to keep up. The doctors were out of options, and the oncologist was bluntly honest—further treatments would not change the timetable much and would only make him sicker. He estimated Jonathan had perhaps three months to live, and hospice care had commenced.

The number struck hard. There had always been some option, some way to fight, some openness in the path ahead. But three months? The reality of this finality was still sinking in for him and Rebecca and for their children—and now for me, too.

Yet there Jonathan was in his garden. He pointed out the carefully marked rows that appeared to be only furrowed dirt. On closer inspection, there were tiny sprouts that promised to be carrots and corn and potatoes. His cabbage, cauliflower, and broccoli plants were coming along well. Jonathan was planting a garden that he knew would outlive him. Yet he was not living in denial; he was simply living. He always told me he wanted to be busy living rather than busy dying.

Planting a garden is always an act of hope. And Jonathan's a man full of hope. Despite this hard news, despite this sudden narrowing of the valley of the shadow of death, he knew he

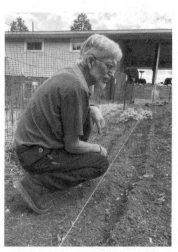

Jonathan in his garden

had a hope that would outlast his cancer. Even as he pulled weeds, Jonathan told me plainly, quoting from Job, "'For He performs what is appointed for me'" (Job 23:14 NASB 1995).

Jonathan told me he hoped to live long enough to cut the first head of cauliflower. In years past, that was always a milestone moment in summer gardening. He and I had often marveled at the cauliflower's fresh white color and magnificent symmetry of form and pattern. Jonathan and

84

I would give praise to the Creator of cauliflower—then divide it and eat it raw on the spot! If we lived to share the first cauliflower this summer, its taste would be bittersweet.

## May 14

When I went by, Jonathan was out in his carport replacing the water pump on his car. He wasn't driving much now, but someone else in his family would need it, so he was doing what he could to keep the car going. He joked that he doesn't have "can't-cer"—he has "can-cer"—so he focuses on what he *can* do rather than on what he *can't* do.

As usual, he worked fast with wrenches and ratchets, and I was useless other than to bring coffee and to try to get him to take a break. We talked about all the road trips we had made together. We often took long trips together when a weekend church meeting in a distant state gave us the opportunity to hit the road. He would say, "I can't preach, but I can drive," so that was our division of labor. It was a great kindness to me. Conversation, coffee, music, and the ever-changing countryside kept us going. Being a skilled baker (and an early riser), Jonathan sometimes made cinnamon rolls before we set out at sunrise. They were still warm from the oven—and when the aroma overtook us, we stopped and broke out the thermos of coffee and feasted along the roadside. I have sermon notes that are stained with sticky goodness!

I told Jonathan I had another trip coming up later in the summer and perhaps we could set out again. He smiled and agreed we should try.

Tonight I received a birthday present—a collection of Wendell Berry's poems. Surprisingly, the very first one I read reminded me—too much—of that conversation with Jonathan:

> My old friend, the owner
> of a new boat, stops by
> to ask me to fish with him.

and I say I will—both of us
knowing that we may never
get around to it, it may be

years before we're both
idle again on the same day.
But we make a plan, anyhow,

in honor of friendship
and the fine spring weather
and the new boat

and our sudden thought
of the water shining
under the morning fog.[4]

Jonathan and I—in the enthusiasm of the moment—made a hopeful, wishful, impossible plan. Yet, "in honor of friendship and the fine spring weather," we made it anyway.

### May 21

A cold, misty morning. Went over early to sit with Jonathan. He had a recliner brought into his basement study. His two sons had devised a sound system that loops through perhaps a hundred albums of classical music from Jonathan's collection, and also set up new soft, ambient lighting. The routines of day and night were beginning to give way to the rhythms of pain, so now anytime—day or night—he could retreat there in his restlessness.

This morning he had already been there since the dark hours before dawn. He was in his corner recliner, and his orange cat, Bella, was curled up on his lap. After coffee, Jonathan wanted to show me the progress of his garden. The cabbages, broccoli, and potatoes were loving the cool, wet weather and were starting to crowd their rows. We walked a row or two, and Jonathan cut a head of broccoli for me the size of a softball. But all of this was exhausting for him, so we went back to his quiet corner, where a Mozart concerto whispered from the other side. There were shelves stuffed with Jonathan's well-read books, plaques, assorted souvenirs, and an array of family pictures that ranged from his grandchildren to his grandparents—a mosaic of his life that seemed to be fading in the faint light.

We talked a lot about gratitude, and Jonathan said something that was surprising to me about the liberating power of God-given gratitude for a God-given affliction. He said, "I'm not glad I have cancer, but God has given me enough of a glimpse into this thing to realize it's not about cancer. That frees me to be able to sit back and enjoy so many associated blessings—blessings we would never enjoy otherwise. Do you think Shakespeare was afflicted and therefore enabled to write 'Sweet are the uses of adversity'?"

I admired one of the pictures nearest him. It was one of his wife, Rebecca, when they first met and married. Jonathan unfolded the story for me of how they met. He spoke with wonder about how *he* got to marry *her*, and the sacred mystery of how they had been kept for each other. In all the world and the others they had known, on a certain day their paths crossed— and then they became one. Jonathan was smitten from the beginning—and he still is.

Something had been nagging at Jonathan almost since his cancer diagnosis over two years prior. He has brought it up to me several times before, and he told me he had had a sudden revelation. He said that near the beginning of his journey with metastatic cancer someone gave the book *Joni & Ken: An Untold Love Story* to Rebecca—only he scooped it up and read it first. Joni Eareckson Tada wrote about her own battle with cancer,[5] but there was something she shared that Jonathan didn't quite know what to do with: "Cancer hadn't felt like a gift in the beginning. No, not at all."[6]

Jonathan said, "That line grabbed my attention because the inference is that she came to see cancer as a gift. I thought about that and found it amazing. I remember thinking that I wasn't there. I didn't see cancer as a gift, nor was I thankful for it. This didn't trouble me because we read the verse 'Be thankful in all things,' and we concluded that being thankful IN something is different from being thankful FOR something. So I wasn't convicted about my gratitude condition because I felt that I was thankful and that's as far as that needed to go. A couple of weeks ago I was musing, and my musings went something like this: *I'm thankful for cancer because it has allowed me to see facets of my wife's godliness that I might have missed otherwise.* As soon as I thought that, I was shocked. What did I just say? That was one of those moments! To be thankful for cancer had never been my goal, and yet God reached down and touched my heart to show me that it is possible even for me to be thankful for cancer: gratitude to God for cancer, gratitude for Rebecca in the cancer, gratitude for our marriage."

Despite this painful twilight path they were walking together, these two could still find things to laugh about. Jonathan told me that a few weeks back, as he was taking some of his meds (he has a dizzying array of dosages and combinations and times for them to be taken that it practically takes a pharmacist to keep track of it all), Jonathan got some of the medicine mixed up and took the wrong ones. He quickly realized his mistake and, flustered, asked Rebecca, "What do you think is going to happen?" Without missing a beat, she said with a hint of a smile in her eyes, "You could die." Then they started laughing. Jonathan was still laughing as he recounted that moment when his brave, God-trusting wife could laugh in the face of death. And Jonathan loved her all the more for such courage.

### June 9

Rebecca had to be away, so I went over to be with Jonathan. Despite his protests to the contrary, he really shouldn't be left alone. When I arrived just after seven o'clock, he had already been up since four—weary hours governed by pain rather than by the clock. The daily doses of morphine helped, but murmurs of pain still slipped out in a kind of unconscious groaning. The cancer in his bones was particularly agonizing, and he had to stay ahead of its stabs.

We had coffee along with some fresh granola his daughter Jo had just made. Jonathan's granola is well-known among those blessed to know about it and would leave the best chef drooling with envy. The fragrance of toasted oats, coconut, walnuts, dried cherries, and apricots with a hint of honey and cinnamon still lingered in the air. As we tucked into it, he took a mighty pride in telling me how he taught Jo to make it. It's his gift to her that will truly keep on giving! And the fact that the original recipe had been lost years ago only added to the mystique of the measures.

We went out to the garden for a bit. Less and less could he go to his backyard garden, but he told me it is a place he goes to be alone, to cry, and to stifle his sobs. Jonathan wanted to water some of the plants in his greenhouse, but the effort was exhausting and the midmorning sun too hot, so we went back to his quiet corner in the basement.

Jonathan kept books of puzzles handy—they helped keep his mind distracted from the pain. He's a tenacious Sudoku puzzler, but this morning it was crosswords. Now and then he kept me in the loop as he filled in answers. Googling—the bane of the brain—is *not* allowed in word puzzles! But asking a friend is perfectly permitted!

Jonathan asked, "House of Lords members?"

"Peers."

"Ljubljana resident."

"Slovenian."

"Too many letters."

"Slovene?"

"Yes!"

Several minutes passed as he crossed off more questions. Then he asked, "River through Warsaw." We had both crossed that river in our past travels in Poland, but now we both drew a blank. Jonathan was drifting off in his recliner, while Bach and Beethoven played quietly in the other corner. Now and then the click of his pen strokes on the page revived, then slowed, until his hand—pen in hand—slipped from the page. As he slept, his hand occasionally took on the motion of writing, as if he had remembered the name of the river.

### June 23

Jonathan was so weak, so thin—his sagging clothes stretched over his gaunt frame. We had coffee at the table. His once-strong, large, quick hands inured to hard work now trembled to steady a cup. He could take only a few sips, then went back to his bed. He was no longer able to go down the stairs to his favorite corner and recliner, so a hospital bed provided by hospice would have to do. He settled in, and I slipped my chair up close because his voice had grown so faint. The painful bone cancer in his rib cage and the now unchecked ravages of cancer in his lungs were literally taking his breath away. I leaned in, and he said with a sigh, "My bones are getting so tired."

But his mind was clear. Though I asked him to just ignore me and rest and I'd just sit there in case he needed anything, he wanted to talk. With his usual sense of humor, Jonathan called hospice "his retirement," and with a fleeting smile he added, "Like a rich man, at age fifty-nine, I've been able to retire early." There was not a trace of bitterness in his voice. He knew he was about to gain a princely inheritance. Yet there was sorrow at leaving his Rebecca, their children, and their two sweet grand-daughters, who will likely only know him through pictures.

Though Jonathan couldn't speak beyond a whisper, we talked for more than an hour. We recalled together the beginnings of our friendship nearly twenty years before. I told him soon we were going to part ways for a time. "You are crossing the river." I told him he had been such a faithful brother to me. Even as the dark waters gathered at his feet, my friend never failed to point me to Christ and reminded me often that our God is always and only good. Jonathan said, "Either God is sovereign or He isn't—not almost, or over this but not over that." Then, gathering all the breath his tattered lungs could muster, he raised his voice in praise, "God *is* sovereign! He is!"

### July 1

Went to see Jonathan. He could no longer get out of bed or talk much anymore. When I came in and took his hand, he recognized me and said something, but his words were just whispers. I'm sad I couldn't understand what he said. We held eye contact, and I assured him I was going to simply sit next to him, sip my coffee, and he needed only to rest. With a faint smile, I could tell he understood. He settled back and drifted into an agitated sleep. From time to time I gripped his hand to remind him I was still there.

Spurgeon said, "Friendship is one of the sweetest joys of life. Many might have failed beneath the bitterness of their trial had they not found a friend."[7] Jonathan had always been that kind of friend to me. I hoped in a small way I could be that kind of friend to him now.

I remembered last year, near the beginning of my own cancer journey, I had a biopsy surgery in Bethesda, Maryland. That morning, Debbie and I walked the mile from my hotel to check in to the hospital at five-thirty. It was dark and cold and misting—a miserable morning for a surgery that loomed large with question marks. As Debbie and I trudged along the dark street, my phone buzzed. It was a text from Jonathan:

"My sheep hear my voice, and I know them, and they follow me; and I give eternal life to them, and they will never perish; and no one will snatch them out of my hand. My Father, who has given them to me, is greater than all; and no one is able to snatch them out of the Father's hand. I and the Father are one."[8]

I'm praying for you both this morning. It's another day for renewal of the inner man.

Jesus had just said in this chapter, "I am the good shepherd. . . . I lay down my life for the sheep. . . . No one takes it from me, but I lay it down of my own accord. I have authority to lay it down, and I have authority to take it up again" (John 10:14–18). And soon He would prove it! It is this almighty Jesus who said of His people, "They will never perish; and no one will snatch them out of my hand" (John 10:27 NASB1995).

I still laugh for joy to remember that moment of awe, that wonder, over such a strong Rescuer—and how that text message stopped me in my tracks on a miserable morning in Maryland! In the middle of the battles Jonathan and I were both in, my friend shouted encouragement from his foxhole to mine, "Look at our strong Shepherd. Look at our Captain!"

As I sat by Jonathan's bed in the dim light with the oxygen machine humming along indifferent to his pain, I knew a glorious reality was at work. Now the Shepherd-King, that strong Captain with scarred hands, was carrying His beloved Jonathan in His arms to be with Him forever.

**July 4**

Today Jonathan crossed the river. By the time I reached his side, he was already far beyond all of us. Outside, the sky darkened and a sudden storm opened up. At first, I thought the heavens—like my heart—were weeping. Then I remembered the back-yard garden. It seemed to me that Jesus, who Himself was once thought to be a gardener, was saying, "Well done, good and faithful servant," as the rain washed over all of Jonathan's hopeful planting.

# KNEE-DEEP IN WONDERS

> We say, then, to anyone who is under trial, give Him
> time to steep the soul in His eternal truth. Go into the
> open air, look up into the depths of the sky, or out upon
> the wideness of the sea, or on the strength of the hills
> that is His also; or, if bound in the body, go forth in the
> spirit; spirit is not bound. Give Him time and, as surely
> as dawn follows night, there will break upon the heart
> a sense of certainty that cannot be shaken.[1]
>
> —Amy Carmichael, *Gold Cord:*
> *The Story of a Fellowship*

Look at your fish" was essentially the entrance exam that
the famed nineteenth-century naturalist Louis Agassiz
required of his freshmen students at Harvard. The price of
admission was steeper than it might sound. Samuel Scudder,
one of Agassiz's students, recalled his professor's seemingly
strange test. Agassiz would take a dead fish from some foul-
smelling jar on his shelf and then tell the student to "look at
your fish." Scudder, who would go on to become America's
leading entomologist, described what would become one of
the most important lessons in his life:

> In ten minutes I had seen all that could be seen in that fish. . . .
> Half an hour passed—an hour—another hour; the fish began

to look loathsome. I turned it over and around; looked it in the face—ghastly; from behind, beneath, above, sideways, at three-quarters view—just as ghastly. I was in despair.

I might not use a magnifying glass; instruments of all kinds were interdicted. My two hands, my two eyes, and the fish: it seemed a most limited field. I pushed my finger down its throat to feel how sharp the teeth were. I began to count the scales in the different rows, until I was convinced that that was nonsense. At last a happy thought struck me—I would draw the fish, and now with surprise I began to discover new features in the creature.[2]

After a few hours, Agassiz returned to inquire what the student had learned. It wasn't nearly enough, and the professor told him to keep looking. Scudder recalled:

I was piqued; I was mortified. Still more of that wretched fish! But now I set myself to my task with a will, and discovered one new thing after another. . . . The afternoon passed quickly; and when, toward its close, the professor inquired: "Do you see it yet?"

"No," I replied, "I am certain I do not, but I see how little I saw before."[3]

The exam lasted for three days. Scudder reported discoveries along the way, but always the professor's response was "Keep looking." Young Samuel came to see that Agassiz's exhortation to "Look at your fish" wasn't just an odd freshman initiation—it was the door to discovery through keen and continuous observation.

Agassiz's simple lesson reminds me of how my friend Julie Zickefoose has taught me to look and listen—not in a classroom experiment but in this whole wide world, beginning in the half-acre world of my own backyard.

Cancer has awakened more delight in what's in front of me rather than just what's ahead of me. Much of my life has been about going on to the next thing, then the next thing, then the next. But my present days are precious, so I want every sense of mine to be awake to what's right before me. "This is the day that the LORD has made; let us rejoice and be glad in it" (Psalm 118:24) is more than a sanctified slogan—it's an invitation to take joy in what God has made.

In the suffering and uncertainty of this journey, I've found more joy in my marriage, in my morning reading and prayer, and in the company of old friends. I've also found more delight in the little things that surround me—the coffee I'm having now as I write, the clouds that slip above me promising rain, listening to the cicadas that make their siren call from the great oak next to our back porch, and watching a tireless pair of bluebirds come and go from their nest, making more babies before the summer's done.

In God's kindness, my friendship with Julie began at the very beginning of my cancer journey. My conversations with her and visits to her corner of Appalachian Ohio deepened my wonder of the creation and, therefore, of the Creator. Julie is a leading ornithologist who can open up the bird world to others because she's an artist, an author, and—in her words—a woodswoman. I've always loved birds and trees and flowers, but Julie's keen eyes and ears matched with deep knowledge of all things on the wing or in the woodlands opened the door even wider to this world. And in all of it, I see the majesty and the mystery of God's design. If we look, we can see His fingerprints everywhere—from the stained-glass wings of a monarch butterfly to the migratory path of the ruby-throated hummingbird, which can cross the Gulf of Mexico in a single day. The Master's brushstrokes are in all of these things.

But God's design isn't seen only in pretty things or in stunning facts. His design is also in my life—in the things that make sense and in the things that don't make sense. His plan is unfolding whether I'm chasing butterflies with dear friends

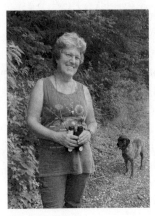

Julie Zickefoose

or walking this hard path of cancer. My God, the God of wonders, has designed it all, and I'm learning, ever so slowly, that His grace and goodness do not stop with the reach of my understanding or comfort.

David, my friend of thirty years and a pioneer in the Gospel's advance in the Balkans, was back home and planning a trip to Ohio. In hitching a ride with him, I saw the perfect convergence of opportunities—the chance to spend time with David and to introduce him to Julie. Together we would have a delightful day with her. I knew she would take us into the woods and meadows and help us look—and look some more—until we saw how little we had seen before.

### Indigo Hill
### July 14, 2022

After a restless night—more like intermittent naps—I awoke as the sky was pinking the east. In the spare light, Julie's meadow was like a dark sea rolling all the way to a tree line that framed the dawn. It was too early to face the day, so I slept another hour—maybe two. When I got up, the house was surprisingly quiet. David was still sleeping, and Julie's son, Liam, had already left for work. I went out to find Julie and to greet the day. The sun had cleared the tree line, and Julie was walking up from the garden with a basket of freshly picked beans. Her feet were wet with dew, and her faithful brindle dog, Curtis, trailed behind. The sun was quickly warming the day, and the meadow that I could only make the faintest outline of by the dawn's early light was now a wide, undulating field of prairie grasses and flowers fresh with dew—a thick tangle of life already humming with katydids and cicadas.

We went in for breakfast with David and talked over the day ahead. Julie had kindly cleared her schedule so we could have this day together to explore. She normally has correspondence and editing work for the bird-watching magazine *BWD* or has commissions to paint. And there's the maintenance and care of this place. Julie lives on an eighty-acre sanctuary called Indigo Hill, and since the death of her husband to cancer three years ago, it falls to her to care for it.

In these summer months, the mowing of the yard and meadow paths alone is a big, ever-growing job in itself. Julie has had a lot of trouble with her riding lawnmower this summer. Last week, after getting the mower back from the repair shop, she got right to work—but she wasn't at it five minutes before the blade stuck fast into a root. Julie had to dig out the root and saw it off the blade before proceeding. That kind of grit and drive characterizes her life and work in so many ways, whether she's saving an orphaned blue jay, rescuing an injured hawk, protecting a beaver habitat from poachers, or caring for her family and friends.

Julie decided there were wonders enough to see on Indigo Hill, so we wouldn't go on our long rambles through the woods as we once did. I think she sensed I'm too weak for that now but is too kind to say it, so she, David, and I went out into the big meadow along a wide path that wound through it. The prairie grasses and flowers were shoulder high all across, except for the gray-headed coneflowers, which looked down on us from seven feet up. Good rain this summer fed this lush field and spattered it with blossoms of yellow, purple, and pink.

As we walked along, a sharp *cuk-cuk-cuk* sounded from the woods. It was the staccato call of a big pileated woodpecker, and we heard other birds call from deeper in the forest. Julie

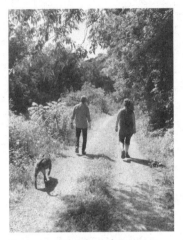

Exploring with Julie and Curtis

said they were indigo buntings. Her ear is always pitch-perfect to about every species of bird-call in this hemisphere! As we walked on, more calls and piping sounds could be heard. "White-eyed vireo," Julie said with a hint of hushed wonder, as if she were hearing this call for the first time instead of the thousandth time. There are a dozen kinds of warblers that come and go on Indigo Hill, but Julie can separate out all of their songs. Whether it was the buzzy sound of the blue-winged warbler, which nests in these grasses, or the whistle of the indigo bunting, whose tune sounds like *sweet-sweet-too-too*, she kept a running record of who was calling. Julie said to me, "It's not just noticing—it's caring and truly wanting to know the name of each creature, how it makes its living, how it fits into that bigger web woven all around me in this humming, creaking, chirping meadow."

Birdsongs mingled with the buzzing-sizzling sounds of this gorgeous grassland, for the meadow is an incubator of life for every kind of bird, bug, and butterfly, along with an assortment of snakes and box turtles. I was not prepared for such beauty. The colors of the meadow against the brilliant sky were a sight to behold, but it was the music of the meadow that stopped me in my tracks. It reminded me of C. S. Lewis's story of how Aslan created Narnia:

> The Lion was pacing to and fro about that empty land and singing his new song. It was softer and more lilting than the song by which he had called up the stars and the sun; a gentle, rippling music. And as he walked and sang the valley grew green

with grass. It spread out from the Lion like a pool. It ran up the sides of the little hills like a wave.[4]

And today, from this bright land, the creatures sang in antiphony to their Creator. As the psalmist said, "Let the fields be jubilant, and everything in them; let all the trees of the forest sing for joy" (Psalm 96:12 NIV).

On the far side of the meadow, the path took us into the woods of an old orchard. There were remnants of fruit trees, but mostly it's all grown over with tulip trees, dogwoods, spicebush, and persimmon trees—a favorite tree of mine—which are straight as an arrow. In fact, persimmon wood makes good arrow shafts, and its fruit in season makes a tasty woodland snack.

Our path through the old orchard eventually opened up into another smaller meadow. What the orchard meadow lacked in size it made up for in exuberance. As we walked up, a flock of goldfinches shot up from the thick tangle like sparks from an anvil. Julie said they were feeding on the seeds of the coreopsis, whose yellow blossoms ran through the meadow like veins of gold. There was so much color—purple coneflowers, pink milkweed, black-eyed Susans, the orange tops of butterfly weed, and delicate blue bergamot, which tiger swallowtails lingered over, indifferent to our closeness.

Julie has a bench at the edge of the meadow that she calls her "office." I sat there for a while as she and David walked about the meadow. Julie regaled him with stories of the turkeys, deer, and bobcats that also walk these paths in their turn. Julie's office was a pleasant place in the meadowland to rest and write. Amid this lush life, I couldn't help but recall lines from the old poem "Knee-deep in June." There I was "knee-deep" in wonders, and feeling as laid back as the Hoosier farm boy in James Whitcomb Riley's sonnet to summer.

TELL you what I like the best—
    'Long about knee-deep in June,
    'Bout the time strawberries melts
    On the vines—some afternoon
Like to jes' git out and rest,
    And not work at nothin' else!

Orchard's where I' ruther be—
Needn't fence it in for me!
    Jes' the whole sky overhead
      And the whole airth underneath—
      Sorto' so 's a man kin breath
    Like he ort, and kindo' has
Elbow-room to keerlessly
    Sprawl out len'thways on the grass,
      Where the shadows thick and soft
As the kivvers on the bed
    Mother fixes in the loft
Allus, when they's company!

Jes' a sort o' lazein' there—
    S' lazy, 'at you peek and peer
      Through the wavin' leaves above,
      Like a feller 'ats in love
And don't know it, ner don't keer!
Ever'thing you hear and see
    Got some sort o' interest. . . .[5]

*Everything* has some sort of interest! That's exactly how I feel right now. Julie recently wrote an article in *The Wall Street Journal* and noted that we can see only 1 percent of the colors a bird can see.[6] Even though we share the same planet, birds evidently see the world in colors we can't even imagine. But though I lack a bird's eye view, I've made the most of my 1 percent this morning! There's so much to see—and the more I look, the more I see. And the more I listen, the more I hear.

The sun rose higher, and so did the heat; we went in for lunch, and afterwards, Julie used the hottest part of the day to paint. She's closing in on completing a commission for an ornithological society. The watercolor is of a Wilson's warbler in flight over the Maine coast. An eclectic playlist runs while Julie paints, and she often joins in singing backup with her favorite bands. Julie has a great voice and was at her best today singing "Jolene" with Norah Jones and was in sync with J. D. Souther on "New Kid in Town," all while mixing and brushing on the warbler's correct colors.

I used the studio time to learn more of Julie's backstory. My friend is a Harvard-educated ornithologist, a writer, an artist, and all-around tour guide to Creation—but where did her love for birds and growing things begin? Julie told me growing things got in her blood from nursery school, when she and her fellow classmates were given paper cups with petunia seeds that they grew in the windowsill of the classroom. She said the day she brought her purple petunia home in that paper cup was like carrying the holy grail.

When Julie was eight years old, she was exploring the woods near her home, which included some wetlands. As she followed the squirrels and chipmunks, she heard a fluttering sound in a pool of water. Julie told me she dropped down on her knees and crawled under a patch of briars so she could see what was making the sound, and there in the pool was a blue-winged warbler flashing its brilliant gold and blue feathers in the water. Julie's first thought was, *Is this a fairy?* There, crouched beneath the briars, she had her first life-changing connection with the bird world.

Julie's paintings have graced covers of some of the best magazines and books of the birding world, including the books she's written. As she brushed on the wings of a warbler in flight, I asked her how she learned to paint. Julie said drawing or painting birds was just another way of studying them more intensely.

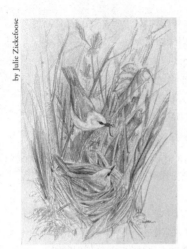

by Julie Zickefoose

Blue-winged warbler

Then when she was sixteen, she went to a summer art camp. In her words, "It was a camp for students who weren't afraid to be excellent, kids who weren't too cool for school." One of the teachers in the camp was an accomplished artist who saw Julie's talent, and he gave Julie a list of materials needed for his painting class. She said her mom swallowed hard at the cost but made the investment in the brushes, paints, and expensive paper—and Julie took it from there!

Julie's dad was a big influence as well and encouraged her to explore and learn about life in the outdoors. She said what she most admired about her father was his encyclopedic knowledge. He was always investigating something and would go to the library and bring home a giant stack of books—and then would sit at the dinner table and "hold forth," excitedly sharing whatever he was currently discovering. It could be something historical, mechanical, or natural. Julie said, "I'm always looking for my dad—people like him who know things because they are reading, doing, and inventing."

Early evening, Julie prepared dinner, and we ate outside near the big meadow. She made roast pork seasoned with rosemary, garlic, and brown sugar along with sweet potatoes and the green beans from the garden this morning. Liam, David, and I all enjoyed it immensely—but Curtis was especially happy with the pork bone Julie gave him, and he took it away to a favorite spot where he could gnaw and crunch in perfect peace. Julie also made a peach cobbler from some just-picked peaches that Debbie sent up for her. It made for a fine finish!

We watched and heard the meadow in twilight. A yellow-throat stood sentinel over the footpath we took through the meadow that morning, and the warbler sang his evensong along with other birds deeper in the field—their voices dying with the day. But soon, their calls were taken up by the night creatures, who continued the chorus, for the meadow never sleeps.

Just as the sun was setting, we witnessed the opening of the evening primroses. We brought our chairs up close so we could catch every moment of this twilight wonder. The yellow blossoms start closed like a parasol until sunset. Then one by one, by the score, they open up in their full glory. If you listen closely enough, there's a little *thh-wip* sound and a puff of fragrance when the bloom springs open.

Joining us for the grand opening were large Pandorus sphinx moths. These green and pink beauties make a shuttering sound when they fly, like an old crop duster coming in for a landing. The moths, drunk with nectar, kept up their teetering flight from one primrose to the next. When I cupped my hands in front of a flower, I could feel their nearness in the gathering darkness. Sometimes—this was the sweetest thing—I could even feel the breath of their wings on my cheek as more flew in for the feast.

After the primroses were all opened, we left them to the Pandorus sphinxes, which by now could be heard but not seen in the deepening dusk. We took our chairs back around to the meadow for the moonrise and to watch the fireflies dance in the dark. Julie said there are five different species of lightning bugs there, and the ones we watched are called "Big Dippers" because of the way their light trail makes a *J*. Amazing. I never knew God made so many kinds of fireflies! Whether in the great things or the smallest things, Lord, I praise you, for "you are the God who works wonders" (Psalm 77:14).

I'll never forget that summer evening. The full moon slipped through a veil of clouds and spilled silver light over the meadow. We talked and laughed until it was late, our faces washed in moonshine as the crickets and katydids sang over us.

# THE DAY THE WALLS
# CAME DOWN

Something there is that doesn't love a wall, that wants it down.[1]

—Robert Frost, "Mending Wall"

We live in a world of walls, and the ones I seem to see most these days are the walls of hospitals and doctors' offices. Their drab paint and fluorescent-faded prints seem like the perfect décor for such walls. However, even if they were painted in posh colors and decorated like a gallery in the Louvre, they would still hem me in a place whose only reward is escape. Like a perpetual return from daylight savings time, it seems like the clock is always going backwards. My frustration with these walls of waiting is far more than loss of control over my days as I go from one appointment to another. The deeper frustration is that cancer forces me to wait on my future as I stare at the broken clock of my present and wonder when the door of my future will open again. I try to be a good patient—I really do—but even the word *patient* implies a forbearance I do not possess. But I know

God can bring down these walls of waiting because I've seen Him bring down far more imposing walls—and I am asking Him to do just that.

A formative event of my life was during a trip to eastern Europe as the Iron Curtain was parting. The literal and political walls of Communist control had penned in whole nations, and the bristling symbol of this oppression was the Berlin Wall. It was a hundred miles long and cut through the heart of Berlin, surrounding its western half to divide the Communist east from the democratic western side of the city. Over time, minefields, barbed wire, sandpits, and guard towers were added to the concrete barrier in order to prevent escape. Even still, thousands risked crossing the wall to freedom in the West—and hundreds died trying—before the God who brought down the walls of Jericho brought down this wall, too.

By the time I was in Berlin, the Wall was just piles of broken concrete waiting for the landfill. I fished out a large chunk of it and tucked it into my backpack. In the weeks ahead, as I continued by train and foot across Europe, my back would regret my greed in getting such a big piece of the wall. But today, as I pen these lines, it sits on a shelf before me. It's a constant reminder that the One who "fixed all the boundaries of the earth" (Psalm 74:17) can move or remove any of them. It's His place—all of it.

There are other kinds of walls—not of the Berlin or Jericho kind—but walls of fear, walls of unbelief, walls of comfort. These walls, brick by brick, rise unseen around us, held together by mortar of our own making. God can bring these walls down, too. I saw that in Greece when I spent time among some extraordinary Christians in the ancient and modern city of Athens. The walls of their church had become blinders to their city, but God would use the most unlikely events to open their eyes. I will never forget the courage and compassion of those Christians—and though I didn't know it then, the timing of my visit was appointed by my loving God. While on that trip, I noticed it was painful for me to walk—and a number of months later I would learn the pain was because of cancer. In the time since my diagnosis, the lessons I learned in Athens have steadied me as I remembered how amid the blood, sweat, and tears of Kingdom advance, glory mingled in our days and shone in the faces of those believers in Athens because God was with them. He is always enough, and I needed to see that at the outset of my cancer journey.

Here's the story of how the walls came down in Athens and what happened afterwards.

### Athens, Greece
**September 7, 2018**

There is a church in the heart of Athens that has been a faithful, Gospel-preaching church for the last 160 years. First Greek Evangelical Church sits within sight of the Acropolis, and I love the unique physical and spiritual connection found in the proximity between where Paul preached and where Pastor Giotis Kantartzis preaches every Sunday at First Church. This Greek brother is joyful and passionate, and it was a delight to have a good chat together in the sanctuary. Giotis told me of the time ten years ago when Athens was convulsed with riots that exploded out of the Exarchia district—a lawless no-go zone for the police just a few miles away. The street outside the church was one of the places where police and protesters clashed. When Giotis heard what was going on, he rushed to the church. When he got there, the

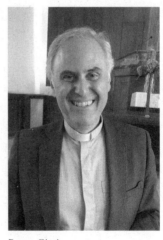

Pastor Giotis

windows were broken and the floor littered with rocks and teargas canisters. He said he began to weep over what he saw. Then, with a smile, he told me he quickly realized it was the tear gas more than the state of the sanctuary that brought tears to his eyes!

The situation calmed down, and the church repaired the windows and went about their business, but subsequent violence out of Exarchia resulted in the windows being broken again—and again. The third time they were broken, Giotis left them that way for a time and used them to point out to the congregation that it was God who was breaking down the walls of their church—their bunker—in order to allow them to see and reach their city. The explosions coming out of Exarchia weren't a call to run and hide. Instead, they were beckoning them to go there with the Gospel of peace. For Giotis and the people of First Church, the riots were a turning point in their following Christ and taking up their cross and running to—and not from—the darkest, hardest places.

Two who answered this call are my friends David and Ruth. David is an American who with joy has come to tell the Good News to people who have not heard. His life is characterized by boldness, endurance, and gentleness. His wife, Ruth, is Iranian and has already lived in four countries, so she knows the life of the wanderer. Besides Greek, she speaks Farsi, Spanish, Italian, and English adorned with a lovely British accent. She is a woman of grace and resilience. Her hands and her table are always open to the outcast, the vulnerable, the unwashed, the hungry, and the broken. Ruth's ministry of mercy is the overflow of the cross-centered mercy of Jesus. She still speaks with joy of the day as a nineteen-year-old when she knew all her sins were forgiven in Christ. In Him she was welcomed, so no matter where she lives, she is always secure, always home.

Their ministry matches this tumultuous city and region, which has seen more than a million refugees pass through over the past four years. More than sixty thousand remain—and more keep coming. These people, fleeing war and poverty, are from the hardest, most closed countries in the Middle East and central Asia: Afghanistan, Iran, Iraq, and Syria. This human wave struck Athens not long after God brought down the "walls" of First Church through the riots and through the grace given to Pastor Giotis. God was preparing them for a great and hard work, and David and Ruth were among those who walked through the breach—and I got to walk with them for a day.

**September 8, 2018**

I walked from the train station early that morning and grabbed a cappuccino on the way to the Acropolis. The city, like me, was slowly waking up, so the coffee helped, as did the brisk walk through the twists and turns of Athens's streets. There's a reason the Greeks invented the word *labyrinth*! But I eventually found a way to a surprisingly quiet shoulder of stone on the edge of the Acropolis, a place known as the Areopagus or—to the Romans—Mars Hill.

In my travels about the Mediterranean, I have often been able to stand among first-century ruins with the book of Acts in hand and say, "Paul was here." But somehow this place was different. Perhaps it's the breeze and blue light of the Aegean morning or the commanding view of the ancient city, but Paul's message of "Jesus and the resurrection" still seems to echo here, as it did in my own heart that morning.

By Paul's time, Athens's glory days were centuries past, but it was still revered as an intellectual capital of the world, filled with philosophers and idolaters. Their shrine to "the unknown god," though, only underscored the fact that all

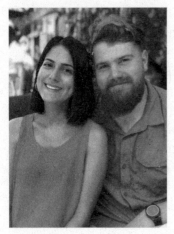

Ruth and David

these smart people did not know it all. In fact, they didn't know the God who made them and all they could see. So there on this hill, Paul introduced the Athenians to their Creator. There could hardly have been a more impressive place for Paul to preach, for rising above Paul was the Acropolis crowned with the Parthenon, the temple to Athena, the city's patron goddess of wisdom. Even in ruin, it's a wonder of the ancient world, but in the first century it was lavished with color and richly appointed with gold and ivory. And beneath Paul, the backdrop was this great city, which stretched to the sea.

My early morning reverie on Mars Hill was broken, though, by the sound of tour buses queuing up below, as well as the pressing demands ahead of me to keep up with David! I went on to find him and Ruth, and we headed to Exarchia to the place known as Integration House. This is the church plant that David and Ruth are a part of, and it's also a place where refugees stay who have nowhere else to go.

I met with the pastors, Tim and Alex. In many ways, the cultural gap these two Greek pastors crossed in moving here from First Church (just five miles away) was as daunting as if they had traversed an ocean. Exarchia is run by anarchists and Marxists and various mafia factions. There are colonies of drug addicts, widespread prostitution, undocumented refugees—and zero churches until this church opened its doors.

A hard step, but a necessary one, was for Alex and Tim to move their families here. Alex said that by living next door to anarchists, they have learned the "right language" to communicate the Gospel to them. But the Gospel first had to do its work in their own hearts. Alex said that they had to repent of their arrogance and ignorance. Just as Christ in His incarnation made Himself of "no reputation," they had to leave the safe zone of their church and community and live in a place where they were nobodies. In the midst of planting a church in this unwelcoming, restless, and occasionally violent place, the city suddenly had a massive influx of refugees from the Middle East. Alex and Tim said the refugee crisis wasn't a distraction. It was part of God's sovereign plan.

Alex pointed out it's easy to quote verses like Deuteronomy 10:19 about accepting the foreigner. But for the Gospel to break through, it had to cost them something. It required identification with the peoples' suffering. Two Kurdish refugees—a pregnant woman and her brother—showed up at the church. They had been sleeping on the streets for weeks and were desperate, but the church at that time had no place to house them. So Pastor Tim gave up his office and let them live there for the next six months until they could be resettled. Another family was so infested with lice that neither the refugee camp nor the hospitals would take them in until they had been quarantined. So Alex and his wife brought the outcasts into their own home.

I was deeply moved by these brothers. I saw Christ in them. I saw Calvary love on display.

Later, Ruth headed to her office, where she counsels and interprets to help refugee women and children get out of the sex trafficking trap, while David and I headed deeper into the graffiti-lined streets of Exarchia. People have painted their gods of rage and lust and despair on the crumbling walls of their world, but there is also an unknown God in Exarchia—one who is making Himself known through His servants. David, Ruth, Tim, and Alex all remind me of what the pioneer missionary C. T. Studd once wrote: "Some want to live within the sound of church or chapel bell; I want to run a rescue shop within a yard of Hell."[2]

David and I went on to a place that is simply called "the squat house." Of course, there are many squat houses—abandoned buildings taken over by squatters—but David and Ruth had recently discovered this one. Spread throughout the eight-story building, more than one hundred undocumented refugees from Afghanistan, Iran, and Syria lived there. They gave all their money to the smugglers who got them to Greece. They couldn't go back, but they also couldn't go forward because they don't have proper documentation to be in Greece. An Iranian believer named Reza, whom David was discipling, helped oversee the squat house, settle disputes, and assess needs. There were now three makeshift showers in the abandoned office building, and David and Ruth were able to provide a gas stove for the squat house.

Besides checking on things, David was also inviting everyone to his apartment the next night so he and Ruth could make dinner for them. He expected about half the people in the squat house to come, so as many as fifty might show up for the feast! David said it was an opportunity to give these people honor by inviting them to share a meal in his home. For many of them, it would be the first time they'd been in a real home in a long, long time.

I followed David and Reza from floor to floor, room to room—many rooms made of no more than sheets strung on clotheslines. On one floor, an Iranian family invited us to share tea and a brown sugar pie called *halva* with them. On another floor, an Afghan family poured out their grief. They had fled Afghanistan four years prior and had been on the move ever since. Their oldest children are twin daughters, but one of them died from exposure during the smugglers' passage across Turkey. The mom, Farzane, held their one-year-old daughter, Mozhghan, in her arms. The sweet little girl with big, wondering eyes had recently been diagnosed with epilepsy, and they feared it was affecting the baby's vision. Farzane and her husband, Sayid, were still reeling from this hard news, and their future is full of fears. She said with tears, "When Mozhghan had her seizure and was rushed to the hospital, David and Ruth were the first family in four years to visit us."

David prayed with them and invited them to his home for dinner the next night. We parted ways and went in search of coffee and some space to make calls. David had a meeting he hoped to make happen. He has been cultivating a friendship with Abul Kalam, the imam of the largest mosque in Athens. David met with him at the mosque a couple of times before, and so he called up the imam to see if he could come by for another chat.

Whoever answered the phone passed it around to several people who were all in bewilderment as to how David would have the imam's number and would know his name. It was amusing to listen as the phone was passed around and hear the awkward silences and side conversations on the other end. Their concerns probably related mostly to their being there illegally, but some mosques are also safe houses for Islamic State terrorists passing through. For example, the ISIS fighters who blew themselves up in France's worst ever terror attack came through Athens before detonating their suicide vests in a crowded Paris soccer stadium. Greece has a reputation as the soft underbelly of Europe for Islamic terror infiltration.[3] For whatever reason, this call from a foreigner was unsettling—but at least they didn't hang up.

Once we knew the imam was in, we didn't ask for an appointment—we just went. The mosque, like many of its adherents we met there, seemed to want to keep a low profile. After a bit of meandering through the makeshift mosque, we met up with the young imam. Abul Kalam is a Bengali, as are most of the men we met. He's a smart guy who can recite the Koran from memory and is proud of his Islamic law library. As we sat in his reading room and talked, a man named Jameel served us ice-cold mango juice and a dish of dates. They showed us much kindness along with a bit of bewilderment.

Friday prayers were soon to be offered, which brought up the subject of how the imam viewed his relationship with Allah. He said he regarded himself as a slave. David gently but plainly contrasted that kind of thinking with his own relationship with God as his Father and how God calls His children sons and daughters.

Preparations at the mosque for the Friday sermon pressed us for time, so David invited the imam to continue the conversation over a meal in his home. Abul Kalam agreed to come, and they exchanged contact information. Before parting ways, the imam showed us the large room where the men pray. The floor had stripes painted on it that were oriented toward Mecca so the men could all bow in good order. The imam doesn't know it yet, but David and I are now praying for him, asking that all the neat little lines of his religion would fall apart beneath the shadow of the Cross and that through Christ, Abul Kalam, the slave of Allah, would become a child of God!

David had one more place to go to that afternoon before we headed back to his apartment. Viktoria Square is a regular part of his ministry circuit each week and is a place well-known to the refugee community, so we headed there. However, we were both hungry, and the snack at the mosque was just an appetizer. On the outskirts of Exarchia we found a quiet café and had delicious baked fish, which looked up agreeably from the platter and was probably pulled from the sea that morning. It was a good time to catch our breath and talk.

I especially wanted to hear how David came to faith in Christ. In John Bunyan's *Grace Abounding to the Chief of Sinners*, he wrote, "It is profitable for Christians to be often calling to mind the very beginnings of grace with their souls."[4] Like Bunyan, David's story is also one of abounding grace.

When David was a teenager, he professed Christ as his Savior, but he had a lot of mixed-up ideas about what being a Christian meant. He enjoyed getting involved at his church and playing drums with the worship band, but he thought of Christianity as something to bless him and meet his needs. It was as if God existed for him. David admitted that he had it exactly backwards.

Another Christian offered to meet with David and study the Bible together. The consistent time in the Word opened this high schooler's eyes more and more to God and the Gospel—and then the storm came. A literal storm. One day David was caught in a terrific thunderstorm with a booming sky and hair-raising cracks of lightning that left him somewhere between fear and awe. David saw how small he was and how big God is. God didn't exist for David. David's life was from God and for God. Romans 11:36 came to David's mind, where it says of Jesus, "For from him and through him and to him are all things. To him be glory forever." That day, beneath that turbulent electric sky, David's world changed. His heart changed.

Moved by what he was learning in the Word and his growing vision of God, David started a Bible study with his high school football team. A number of girls wanted to join in, too, so they started meeting at a frozen yogurt shop. They soon packed the place out, so they added more gatherings as the numbers grew. These gatherings were organic, authentic, and simple—and many were converted as a result.

As our disheveled lunch plates gave way to afternoon coffee before we set out for Viktoria Square, David had one more thing he wanted to share from his story. During the time he was leading the Bible studies, he heard a sermon by David Platt about the more than two billion people who have yet to hear the Gospel even once, and the vast swaths of the world where there are no churches, no Bibles, no Christians. Platt then asked, When would that situation become intolerable for Christians? For David, who had never before heard of unreached people groups, the needs of the Gospel-destitute suddenly became "intolerable." It kept him up at night. He even put pictures of jihadists on his wall in order to focus prayer on the hardest to reach.

On his first trip to Athens, he heard of Afghan, Syrian, and Iranian refugees who spent time in Viktoria Square. He took a backpack of Gospel tracts and went to talk with people there—only to find (to his surprise) that they didn't speak English! David laughed remembering this and said, "I was so naïve." He went on to say of that younger version of himself with his simple, joyful willingness to go anywhere and tell anyone about Jesus, "I miss that boy." However, David hasn't lost that drive, although he has broken the language barrier. And so, David set out yet again for Viktoria Square, and I had the privilege of accompanying him and seeing Calvary love in action.

The plaza is a place of drug trafficking, human trafficking, and sex trafficking—as well as Gospel opportunity. David comes here often to play backgammon. The game is popular with Afghans and Iranians and is a magnet for engaging in conversations. We started a game, and David tried to teach me the basics. Before long, a young Afghan came over to watch. Zamir was unimpressed with my backgammon skills, and I gladly turned the board over to him. David learned that Zamir was a fifteen-year-old refugee from eastern Afghanistan. He had no family there. David told him about the place where Ruth works where he could stay, get back in school, play sports, and develop skills.

Zamir listened but was soon called away by some men. He ran back and told David he would return soon to hear more.

At the end of the square, some men hugged the boy, and they walked off together. Zamir is one of the hundreds of unaccompanied minors who sell themselves for as little as five dollars—exploited by evil men who take advantage of these hungry, desperate kids. As David and I waited for Zamir, we struck up a game with another young Afghan man, but Zamir never returned. We walked the streets looking for him, hoping for one more conversation, one more chance to throw a lifeline his way. My heart ached to find Zamir, but the boy had vanished down a dark street in Athens.

The Gospel work that David and Ruth are doing here is hard, often thankless, and sometimes hated. But there is also genuine joy that salves the wounds of betrayal and lightens long days. I saw such joy in David and Ruth's faces after supper. For more than two years, they'd poured their lives into the life of an Iranian refugee named Ali. Ali grew in his love and obedience to Christ—and then longed to return to Iran and share the Gospel with his family and friends. Just a few months before—at great risk and with great joy—Ali returned to Iran. David continues to disciple him long distance, spending hours on the phone with him to offer counsel and encouragement.

It was fun to listen in on their Skype call with Ali, who was in Tehran and reported that the church he was planting started out with five and had now grown to thirty-two. He went on to say many of them are bold in sharing their faith. At the time, Ali was visiting with family, and the Word was clearly getting out because a nephew got on the call and said excitedly, "Ali has told us about Jesus! Jesus is Lord!"

Every now and then David and Ruth broke away from speaking Persian to share bits of the conversation with me, but even without that I could see the joy that shone in their faces and voices. This is the Gospel that can cross every kind of barrier and border. This is the Gospel of the Risen King that is so good that a refugee goes back to Iran to tell it!

It was near midnight, and the city was quieting down. David and Ruth were off to bed, and sleep beckoned me, too. The day's journey began on Mars Hill and wound through the squalor of Exarchia and into a mosque of a slave of Allah. We ventured into squat houses and squares where the lost and hungry wait, and the journey ended footsore and happy as we heard that the Kingdom has come to another seemingly impossible place. The Gospel that Paul preached on Mars Hill still has power to save, still fuels the endurance that David and Ruth need for these long days, and it's still bright with resurrection hope because Jesus is with them.

# BRAVE MUSIC

By day the LORD commands his steadfast love, and at
night his song is with me, a prayer to the God of my life.

Psalm 42:8

About midnight Paul and Silas were praying and singing
hymns to God, and the prisoners were listening to them.

Acts 16:25

I first met Joni Eareckson Tada when I was in high school—at
least, I met her the way a million others did. When I could
afford it, I made weekly trips to our little Christian bookshop
in my hometown. I remember coming in one day, and on my
way to the commentaries section to look for a good, cheap addition to my library, I saw her book on a floor display. On the
cover was a young blonde at a sketch board holding a pen in her
mouth, and the book was simply titled *Joni*. I was taken with
her courageous story, but at eighteen years old—about the age
Joni was when she broke her neck in a diving accident—I didn't
really understand her. I thought tragedies like what Joni suffered
happened to people who were in the wrong place at the wrong
time—and if they survived, they could only make the best of

121

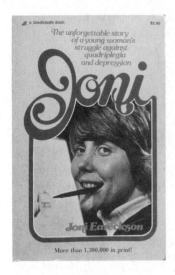

it, as Joni had done. I was slow to understand God's sovereignty and loving purposes in the suffering of His children.

Over the years, Joni's name came up over and over as I traveled— from remote villages in West Africa to ragged stretches of the Middle East. If there was a person in a wheelchair who had any contact with Christians, I usually heard the name *Joni*, regardless of the language spoken. From her wheelchair, Joni was the servant in the parable who brought the broken and discarded ones to a place at her Master's table:

> "Go out quickly to the streets and lanes of the city, and bring in the poor and crippled and blind and lame."
> And the servant said, "Sir, what you commanded has been done, and still there is room."
> And the master said to the servant, "Go out to the highways and hedges and compel people to come in, that my house may be filled."
>
> Luke 14:21–23

When my friend Jonathan was diagnosed with cancer, Joni's name came up again. Her book about her own cancer journey (on top of quadriplegia) strengthened his heart with resurrection hope. And seeing that drew me to read more of her books.

And then, unexpectedly, we met. We were both speakers at a conference in Florida, and between sessions, I spent a delightful day with Joni and her husband, Ken. The most memorable part of the day was just before Joni went on stage to speak. As she prayed backstage, her prayer flowed spontaneously into praise as she led our little gathering in a hymn. It was an unforgettable experience—although I forget the hymn—because right there Joni brought us into the presence of God. And there we worshiped Him.

In early March 2020, I was in Los Angeles and was able to visit Joni. I told her about a book idea I had—to spend a day with different people who had shown me how to live for Christ and journal about that

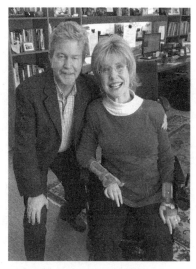

With Joni in Los Angeles, 2020

particular day. I asked if we could spend such a day together, and she readily agreed—yet she warned me, "It won't be very interesting, but there will be lots of singing!" Then I asked her what she'd sung that morning on her way to the office. Her singing is unscripted and spontaneous—the overflow of her love for Jesus—and so she had to think for a minute before her eyes danced and she answered with a rousing refrain of her morning anthem:

> Thine is the glory,
> Risen, conqu'ring Son;
> Endless is the victory
> Thou o'er death hast won![1]

So we made plans to rendezvous again in Los Angeles to spend a day together.

The next day, as I was grabbing lunch in the L.A. airport before my flight home, I overheard two workers at Shake Shack say they'd heard there was a COVID-19 case in the international terminal. I had not heard of a case on these shores before, but it was to be the first drop before the downpour. As everyone reading this knows, the pandemic descended and spread worldwide, turning our lives and plans upside down. Joni, her lungs already fragile from over fifty years as a quadriplegic, was particularly at risk if she contracted COVID. Despite every precaution and safeguard, she still got COVID. It was a close call, but God in His kindness to us brought her through, though the recovery was long and the damage to her tattered lungs lasting.

On my side of the country, a biopsy showed a second, more aggressive cancer, which filled the following months with chemo infusions and sickness. Joni and I tried on three occasions to schedule a day together, strategically tucking it into one of the anticipated "better days" in the rhythms of my chemo schedule. Joni was stronger now and game to make this work, but each time, my situation worsened and we had to postpone.

When I was in the hospital at my weakest point from my cancer treatments, a note came from Joni. Somehow, she always had a sixth sense about when to send the first aid of encouragement and, in her words, "climb into my foxhole and cheer me on." That dark day in the hospital I read this note from her:

*Oh, dear friend, we are praying for you! Borrow this prayer from St. Augustine . . . "God of our life, there are days when the burdens we carry chafe our shoulders and weigh us down; when the road seems dreary and endless, the skies gray and threatening; when our lives have no music in them, and our hearts are lonely and our souls have lost courage. Flood the path with light; we beseech Thee; turn our eyes to where the skies are full of promise; tune our hearts to brave music; give us the sense of comradeship with heroes and saints of every age; and so*

*quicken our spirits that we may be able to encourage the*
*souls of all who journey with us on the road of life, to*
*Thy honor and glory.*"[2]

That prayer took me back to the sacred ground backstage in
Florida when we first met. Joni's heart was tuned to the "brave
music" of seeing and treasuring Christ, even though suffering
so much for so long. Over the years, she has made Christ so
beautiful that others—in a hundred languages of their own—
have joined in the singing.

Joni and I have yet to meet again in person, but we made
the best of it and met via video call and recorded it. It was
another delightful afternoon spent together—only this time
with three thousand miles between us. We talked about her day
and a range of questions. Once during the call Joni became so
overwhelmed that she wept for joy in Christ and in her pain.
The tears just welled up and Joni could not see—and she could
not wipe her eyes. She had to call an assistant and ask her to
wipe away the tears. It was a visible reminder of the limitations she has suffered for over fifty years. It was also a picture
of the glory and grace of God that shall be revealed when one
day He Himself will wipe away the tears from Joni's eyes, and
from my eyes, too—and from the sorrow-stained faces of all
His daughters and sons.

---

**Joni:** *Good to see you, Tim. I cannot believe that you are strong*
*enough, healthy enough, willing enough to do this. God bless*
*you.*[3]

**Tim:** I'm so thankful that we could connect this way, although
it's disappointing that I couldn't come out to see you. It's really
kind of you to open up your day like this and give me some time.

**Joni:** *Absolutely. I can't think of anything I'd rather do today. I've told you this before, but I love your Frontline Missions video series,* Dispatches from the Front. *I've watched them twice, and now I'm on the third time. This time I have a new girl who is helping me at night to give Ken a break. As you know, I have to be turned at night and all these other things. I try and spend that time well and wisely, and so we often listen to audio books. But I told her all about this exciting video series that shows how Christians are advancing the Gospel in some of the darkest places on the earth, and she is so excited to watch them. So, you are a part of the rhythms of my life.*

**Tim:** Praise the Lord. All I'm doing is telling God's story—that's it. It's His story, and His Spirit uses it in people's lives in different ways. And so, it's a blessing to hear that. Thank you so much.

**Joni:** *I so wish you could have spent a day with me out here because I wanted you to meet all the people who help me and see how precious they are and the ministry I have to them—praying for them, their families, and, if they don't know Christ, sharing the Lord Jesus with them. That's such a big part of my life—all the girls who are in and out the front door: hairdressers, moms, retired schoolteachers, women of all different stripes and ages and backgrounds who are such a rich part of the fabric of my life. I'm really sorry you missed that.*

**Tim:** I do wish I could have come and met them and seen your interactions with them. But maybe you can tell me a little bit about them. For example, what is a morning like?

**Joni:** *Usually, it's two girls who get me up in the morning. Many of them do double duty during the week, so they come two or three times a week. They come into the bedroom, turn on* *the lights, stretch my arms. We pray, they give me a bed bath, do my toiletry routines, and get me dressed. Right before I'm ready to sit up, they put on my corset—and we have what we call a corset prayer. It's wearing a corset that enables me to sit up straight and breathe good.*

*So many quadriplegics don't sit up like I do and instead they sit rather slouched and pooched with a distended abdomen, partly because they don't prescribe corsets anymore. I was injured at a time when the rehabilitation philosophy was rather arcane, but I think the corset works—at least it's worked for me for fifty-five years. But it has to be put on expertly to prevent pressure sores and to not exacerbate pain, so we always have a corset prayer. All three of us might pray—or maybe just one of us will—but the corset prayer always includes their family members as well as people who don't know Christ that they're witnessing to.*

*And then, after I am sitting up in my wheelchair, I head to the bathroom, where somebody has to brush my teeth. They feed me breakfast, blow my nose, do all the not so pleasant things. And then, after I'm all finished with lipstick on, we read from Paul David Tripp's devotional. We do that every morning, and sometimes the girls will quickly photocopy a page out of it because David Tripp is so wise. And then we always end with prayer. So it begins with prayer, in the middle is prayer with the corset prayer, then we end with a devotional and prayer.*

*I'm very respectful of their time. When they're done, I say, "Bye. You're late. Get out of here quick." I never want to abuse their kind graciousness, so I try to respect the time that they're here and get them out of here exactly on time. If they need to leave early, I'll say, "Oh, my other friend here, she can pick up the slack. Get out of here, get going. You need to get on with your day." I think they trust me with those responsibilities.*

*And I say thank you a lot—and I mean it. Again, I think of so many quadriplegics that I've met. Some are barely living in developing nations where quads like me normally don't survive. So I just say thank you a lot because I understand the plight of people.*

*To change the subject, where are you in your cancer journey? In your last email you mentioned you have to go through another round of chemo. Is that right?*

**Tim:** I finished the initial chemo: six infusions over the last four months. The next step begins in December, when I start the whole process for the stem cell transplant. The critical phase won't start until January, when I go into the transplant unit for up to four weeks. After I'm released, I'll have about three months of near isolation while my immune system recovers.

**Joni:** *How have you prepared your heart for this? What has helped you face it with such resolved confidence in Christ?*

**Tim:** Honestly, I don't quite know how to prepare. I'm trying to rehearse my hope, spending a lot of time in the Psalms. Earlier today I was going through the passages in John 10, Isaiah 40, and Psalm 23, where we see all the ways in which our Shepherd is not just good, but He's strong. And He's leading the way. I remember how our Shepherd's hands bear the marks of His sacrifice and how He's already gone ahead of us, and He knows the way. I'm just trying to trust Him more.

Sometimes, though, I get these stabs of fear. I don't quite know how to say this because it might sound like I'm bragging, but I normally am not fearful, so this feeling is something I haven't experienced a lot before. But now these stabs of fear unexpectedly strike—kind of like stabs of sorrow. I remember when my mother died of cancer—she's with the Lord now. I preached her funeral, but I never shed a tear until maybe four months later, when the most insignificant thing happened that reminded me of her, and I started crying like a baby.

Like sorrow, fear comes in stabs. I wonder if you could tell me what you think about that? What are your experiences with fear? How do you face fears? I think a big fear I'm facing is there's so much I still want to do, and I feel my life is going to be incomplete. How do I face this? So I'm asking you this big, sprawling question to see what you can tell me.

**Joni:** *Well, I need prayer to answer that, so let me pray. "Jesus, Jesus, Jesus, you hear both Tim and me discussing these things. Both of us suffer in different ways. Neither of us are afraid of death, but it's the dying part. It's the outward man wasting away part that is disconcerting, unnerving, unsettling. And so help me to be as frank and honest as I can in answering Tim's questions, and may our time together be a bolster to both our spirits. May we both be strengthened as you've designed brothers and sisters in Christ to strengthen one another, and to encourage and comfort one another with good words from your words. So help, help us do that, Jesus. Amen."*

*Okay. My fears. Forgive me for the long lapses. It's just that there's so much to say.*

**Tim:** It's a big question. I know.

**Joni:** *I've been down that dark, grim path where fear leads. It's so terrifying and can lead to suicidal despair:* I cannot live like this. I cannot do this anymore. *It was years and years—decades—ago that I felt like that, but the memory of it all is still so real. It's like I can still taste it—it's still so tangible how awful that period in my life was.*

*Now every time fear raises its ugly head, it's like, "Joni, run to God, race to Him, find the cleft in the rock, find the shelter, find the shade of His wings. Park yourself under the shower of His mercies as quickly as you can because you are not going to go down that dark path again."*

129

*Still, fear for me is a daily thing. For example, a helper calls and says, "I'm sorry, my mother called, and I've got to go out of town to help her." That means I've got nobody to help me get up in the morning. I'm always lying in bed when I get that news, so I take a deep breath, embrace that this is of God, and think,* Jesus, this is part of your providential care for me. *Sometimes I see myself as a football being passed off from one person to the next, but I know even if I am dropped by this girl who can't show up because she's got to go tend to her mother's needs, I've got God's everlasting arms underneath me. If it means having to stay in bed, that's okay. I can do this. God is with me. So I try, when I am wedged in the middle of His will, to ease myself there without fear, knowing that this is of the Lord.*

*Fear is so devastating. You can start thinking all kinds of crazy things when you're gripped by fear. I've been down that path before, and I don't want to go there again. But fear comes and raises its ugly head with, for example, what if I break my hip? My bone density is very thin now. I'm a seventy-two-year-old quad, and quads don't even live this long. My lungs are weakened because of COVID. I mean, there are so many things I could be thinking about that could create fear. And like you, I so love what I do. I just so love it. I love talking about Jesus to people with disabilities.*

*For example, the hospital recently called me and said, "We've got a young girl over here who just broke her neck. Would you please come visit her?" How wonderful that a hospital would do that! The administration called me, and they're not even Christians, but they know who I am and thought I could help. So I went over there this week. She and her boyfriend have two children, but he's back in Virginia and could care less. So she's got two little children and a broken neck—and she doesn't know Jesus. She's got ten brothers—none of whom want to take her in—and the hospital's trying to find a care facility to take her. I just sat next to her in my wheelchair, listened to her story, and we cried. I told her, "I just want you to know I feel the weight of what you're going through. And I'm just here."* Tim, I love doing that. I love being there. We have good programs that we do at our ministry (delivering wheelchairs and such), but it's the one-on-one opportunities that I so love. If I couldn't do that, like you, it'd be hard.

So, back to talking about fear. I just ease into what is obviously God's providence for me in my life. Sometimes I get laid up for a while—for example, just two weeks ago I was in bed for about a week with something called autonomic dysreflexia, which is related to my quadriplegia. When that happens, I wonder—is this the shoe that's going to drop? Yikes! But I don't want to go down that dark path. I know I have to stop and take a deep breath, so I start quoting Scripture. I run under the cover of the shadow of His wings. I find that cleft in His rock, and I sing my way through the fear and suffering. I do anything I can, like I said earlier, to get myself back under the shower of God's mercies. I pray, "What can I do, God, to partner with you in moving the ball forward and not back to fear, back to depression, back to anxiety?"

You know, that was really a lot of pancake batter that just spread out on the griddle there, and I didn't have much structure to that response about fear. I was just speaking from my heart.

**Tim:** I know what you mean when you say you can even taste it, the memory of it, and it's a thing not to go back to. I know a little of that—just a little.

**Joni:** *Now my biggest nemesis is chronic pain. Just last night chronic pain jerked me awake. The first thing I do when that happens is look up and see the digital clock display on the ceiling. If it says something like 2:00, then I try to push through the pain and try to breathe my way back to sleep. But if the clock says 4:00 a.m., I know that Jesus has awakened me to* *have communion with Him. Of course, I need more sleep and probably the pain will not subside, but I know there is a more necessary thing. What bolsters my heart, what makes me happy, is to think that I could be one of the early ones rising before dawn to bless Jesus, to think about Him, to fill my chest with Him, to sing to Him, to quote Scripture to Him. Anyway, that helps to keep fear at bay.*

**Tim:** I remember a story you told me, and I wanted to ask you about it today: songs in the night. One of the passages that has meant a lot to me recently is Psalm 42:8: "By day the LORD commands his steadfast love, and at night his song is with me, a prayer to the God of my life." My memory of you in Orlando is how you gathered us and sang and brought us into God's presence. Song led to prayer, and prayer led to song—it was as if it were one. In some ways I think that's what Psalm 42:8 is—"a prayer to the God of my life." So, tell me about songs in the night for you—and maybe even what songs you've sung to Jesus in those four o'clock hours.

**Joni:** *Sometimes I have a hard time putting two words together in prayer because of the mental brain fog of dealing with pain. I just can't get my husband up for the fourth time to prop my pillows some different way. "Try to push my legs forward. Maybe that'll help. Or reposition my hip." I try to limit it to once, at most twice, a night; so I often lay there knowing I'm not going to get back to sleep, and yet I'm in too much pain to really put two words together in prayer. But I can sing hymns.*

*There's something about melody that cooks the sentences together and makes them flow. I don't know much about musicology and why melodies enable you to think sentences in a cohesive stream of thought, but there's something about melodies that do that, and in those night hours, stanzas of hymns will come to my mind easily. Last night I was singing,*

132

All the way my Savior leads me,
Cheers each winding path I tread
Gives me grace for ev'ry trial,
Feeds me with the living bread.

*And I love this stanza:*

Though my weary steps may falter,
And my soul athirst may be,
Gushing from the rock before me,
Lo! A spring of joy I see.[4]

*As I sing these songs, I want to make it my ambition to be pleasing to my Savior, so I'm thinking,* Oh, this must delight you, Lord Jesus. This paralyzed lady in bed with catheters in her and wheezing ventilators singing to you. *I can't really sing out loud because of the ventilator, so I whisper-sing in between the breathing for my lungs, and I think,* Surely you have pity on me. If I were you, I'd have pity on me. I hope this pleases you that out of my weakness, I can demonstrate to unseen powers and principalities. *It's like the Ephesians 3:10 passage, where it says our lives are on display before the unseen world to teach them lessons about God. And so, I am so happy that I get to be His audio-visual aid. And so, I just sing hymn after hymn:*

Jesus, I am resting, resting,
in the joy of what thou art;
I am finding out the greatness
of Thy loving heart.[5]

*I won't bore you—I could go through all four stanzas—but you get the point. I especially love the stanzas of hymns that end on either death or heaven. Like "Rock of Ages," the last verse,*

While I draw this fleeting breath,
When my eyelids close in death,

When I soar to worlds unknown,
See Thee on Thy judgment throne,
Rock of ages, cleft for me,
Let me hide myself in Thee.[6]

*I love those invigorating verses about death and dying and what heaven will be like. But I'm torn—like you are—because I love my work. I love doing what I do, but I would be so delighted to depart to be with Jesus and to see it all come to a conclusion and to leave sorrow and sighing behind us. But the world's broken, so if I can be used to help, heal, restore, and redeem, then keep me moving forward, Jesus. May God heal you and help me so that we can continue to do what we so love doing.*

*So I sing my way through suffering. It's not that I love all this, but it's a Colossians 3 and Ephesians 5 thing. We're not merely invited to sing—we're commanded to sing—and I think God must know that there is something about words and melody together that gives us a unique witness in the creation.*

**Tim:** I remember you told a story in Orlando—and maybe you've written about it before, but it was very precious. You told of a friend who came in and sang to you when you were in the Stryker frame and in despair.

**Joni:** *Oh, I know what you are talking about—it was my friend Sherry. I was very depressed, and she knew it. One night she hiked up the back stairs of the hospital in the middle of the night, long after visiting hours were over. She somehow snuck past the nurses' station and into my room, climbed into bed with me, and snuggled next to me on the pillow. I often describe it like a pajama sleepover. We were just lying there quiet for the longest time, and I was so comforted by her presence. Then she sang,*

Man of sorrows, what a name,
for the Son of God Who came
ruined sinners to reclaim:
Hallelujah, what a Savior.[7]

*And, oh my goodness, it changed me. To this day, I look back on that and can't explain why or how, but she imparted the presence of Jesus and became the embodiment of His grace and goodness to me. In that moment, the nearness and sweetness of my friend was like the nearness and sweetness of Jesus. She made Him real—she made Christ so very real.*

*I often say that people in situations like mine—and like that girl who I just visited in the hospital—we're not always looking for answers. We think we are when we ask "Why?" But we're really looking for somebody to tell us, "Everything's going to be okay, sweetheart." You know, like a little child being lifted up and her daddy patting her on the back saying, "There, there, sweetheart. Daddy's here. It's okay." I resonate with that. We want God to be like that because we want God to be constantly good, and we want Him to say, "Sweetheart, I'm here. Daddy's here. Everything's going to be okay." And answers don't even matter at that point—all that matters is that you believe God is going to make everything okay. No matter what that "okay" pans out to be. It could be pretty brutal for months and even years to come—or as in my case, that I never got healed—but still, He is in the middle of all that. Like Sherry made Him real that night.*

*I often tell people to try not to give people all the biblical reasons why you think God has allowed this to happen in their lives. While those insights might be true, when you're acutely injured, they don't reach where it hurts. They might reach your head, but there are so many emotions going on they don't really help. I just point people to Jesus, who is the answer. He's got all the words.*

**Tim:** I wanted to ask you about your fighting spirit. Whenever I think of Joni Eareckson Tada, I think of a warrior. You have such a tenacity about your life, about your pursuit of God's glory, and about your drive to make Him known to the ends of the earth—all this despite your enormous weakness and limitations.

**Joni:** *Well, I love all that imagery in the Old Testament of God, the Captain of our salvation. "Listen for the rustling in the tops of the balsam trees." It's like a call to arms for me. I'd be the one who, if I joined the army, would say, "Send me to the front lines!" Much like you, I'm sure.*

*I'm driven by the fact that if people with disabilities don't hear about Jesus Christ, the real Jesus, the One who can give them hope in the midst of affliction, they don't hear that their suffering, their disability is only a dark omen of even worse suffering to come in an eternity without Jesus Christ. And man, does that drive me! That's why I get up in the morning. That's why I love what I do. I can't bear to think of the one billion people with disabilities in the world—and you've been around the world, you've seen them—not hearing about Jesus. They are the outcasts, the ones pushed aside. They are non-people. That's what keeps me invigorated. As Paul said to Timothy, I endure hardship like a good soldier. I do not want to shame the Captain of my salvation. A lot of it is that I don't want to shame Jesus. He who went through so much suffering on my behalf. How dare I complain. As Philippians 2:14 says, "Do all things without grumbling or [arguing]." I dare not complain!*

*I remember that the face that Moses longed to see but was forbidden to see yielded Himself to drunken soldiers to be slapped bloody. I often read in Mark where He was led into the praetorium, and the doors closed behind Him where all those drunken soldiers were slapping Him. I think perhaps the Bible is too delicate to say what actually happened behind those* closed doors. *I'm sure they did many more things to Him than we read in print because of the horror of it all. But if Jesus could go through that, I cannot shame Him and cave in. Doesn't mean I won't get depressed. Doesn't mean I won't have times, like David, where I say, "Oh, my soul, why are you downcast within me?" But then the next verse says, "Put your hope in God." It's saying, Come on, put your hope where it needs to be. It's a constant fight, but it really is a good fight.*

*And I don't mean "good fight" in the sense that it has good repercussions or good value. It's good in the sense that it's energizing. It's a good fight in that, when you persevere, you step into this person that you didn't think you were capable of being—and that so energizes you because it's all by the grace of God, it is all Him. It is not me per se. My only role in it is that I'm actively engaged in my own sanctification. I'm ready to say, "Jesus, help me here. I don't want to capitulate." And every time He helps, it's just amazing. You know? And plus, I love esprit de corps—you know, in keeping with the whole warrior theme. I love the esprit de corps with other people with whom I draw strength.*

*I'm not a social media person, but I do have a private Facebook page of thirty-five pain-pals—most of whom I've never met. At least seven of them are totally bedridden and have been for decades. One of them lives in a dark bedroom in Tennessee. She has a strange autoimmune disorder kicked off by Lyme's disease. Anyway, she lives in a very dark bedroom on a mattress on the floor because she's so painfully sensitive to light, sound, and movement. This is our esprit de corps as we constantly post essays, comments, quotes to encourage each other. I don't want to shame my Savior, and I want to be strong for my friends. Not strong in a fake sense. When I say strong, I mean when I can say, "I'm really weak here. I need lots of prayer. I feel myself sinking back down that grim, dark road to depression, and I don't want to go there. Please pray for me."*

*That's the kind of fighting and being strong. I don't mean strong like, "Oh, look at me, I'm on the frontlines. I'm not wavering. I'm not weakening." No, to be strong is to be able to say, "I'm wavering, I'm weakening, but help me, Jesus." And then get others to help you, too. I'm just invigorated by that whole in-your-hardship-as-good-soldier imagery. I love that. It's a call to arms.*

**Tim:** And that esprit de corps imagery is interesting in that it's also a motivation—fighting shoulder-to-shoulder, so to speak.

**Joni:** *Yes, and another's victory is our victory, because we are intimately and intricately linked together mysteriously in the Body. It strengthens me when they persevere—and so I am more able to persevere. I don't quite understand how that works in the body of Christ—that we are one. That we are actually one and that another person's victories become mine, which makes me stronger to fight my own battles. So that whole leaning on others in the midst of your hardships certainly helps.*

**Tim:** I've read enough battle histories to know that wars are largely fought by people who are, when it comes down to it, fighting for their friends.

**Joni:** *You're absolutely right. Like a young man coming back from, say, Afghanistan a few years ago, ready to sign up for another tour of duty for the sake of his friends still over there?*

**Tim:** Friendship in the Kingdom's forward advance is a gift of grace, and I'm so grateful for your friendship. Good friends can also easily while away the hours together, but I want to respect your time.

**Joni:** *Tim, I feel like I've just poured pancake batter out on this griddle. Everything's kind of going everywhere. My answers* and responses haven't been all that well constructed. But I will pray for you with a happy heart, and if there's any way I can serve you, I will jump to it. I will get in your foxhole and do all that I can for you. Let me pray before you go.

Lord Jesus, we are loved with your everlasting love, led by grace that love to know, gracious Spirit sent from you above, you have taught us that this is so. Oh, this full and precious peace; oh, this rapture all divine.

Lord Jesus, thank you, bless you for this time together. And we thank you for the esprit de corps that Tim and I have with one another—and Debbie and my husband, Ken. This esprit de corps that strengthens us as we speak of our own victories in you through our battles, whether they be with quadriplegia, chronic pain, cancer, whatever. Lord Jesus, how good that we can strengthen one another, thank you that you designed your body this way. And, Lord Jesus, I do pray that as this bone marrow procedure is about to take place, I pray for less pain and increased courage and grace.

Father, would you please stretch the capacity for Tim to endure pain? May his pain level capacity be heightened through all of this so that he can absorb it, walk in it, walk through it to the other side and praise you all the more for it. Thank you for Debbie being by his side, his valiant companion, his life partner, his best cheerleader. So Jesus, strengthen her as well. And Father, when their spirits flag, when the tempter tries to beckon them down that dark, grim road to fear and depression, oh God, put up roadblocks: roadblocks from promises in Your Word, roadblocks from favorite hymns, roadblocks of other people's prayers, anything and everything to keep them from falling into discouragement. Lord Jesus, you've ordained our days long before the foundation of the world, so teach us to number them that we might apply our hearts to your kind of wisdom in them and bring healing.

*Most of all, bring hope, and bring Debbie and Tim even closer together. And they've enjoyed obviously a sweet life partnership for many years, bring maybe even closer together. Help them discover even sweeter, more wonderful things to love about each other, and in so doing that this cancer will have not gained a victory but will have been a platform to springboard them both further into a closer, deeper, sweeter walk with you. We love you, Lord Jesus. Oh, do sense how we love you. We love you, Jesus. We just can't do it without you. We're so grateful for our time together. Help Tim to make sense of all this pancake batter. These thoughts blurted and spread out don't seem to make sense to me now as I reflect on them, but as Tim puts them in his note pad—oh, I love his note pad, his journal—help them to make sense so that others might be strengthened. Jesus, we love you. Bless our day. In your name. Amen. Amen. Praise Him, Praise Him ever in joyful song.*

# THE SWEET
# PSALMIST OF TEXAS

If you wait until the conditions are perfect, you'll never write a thing. It's always a matter of the will. The songs won't create themselves, and neither will the books, the recipes, the blueprints, or the gardens.[1]

—Andrew Peterson, *Adorning the Dark*

A few years ago, I was traveling in the Middle East from Arabia to Iraq to Jordan—and then backpacked into Jerusalem. As I set out, a friend shared some songs for the road, an album by Caroline Cobb, who was new to me. The album had captivated my friend by the clarity with which Caroline wrote songs from Scripture. So all along my arduous journey, Caroline kept me company as she opened the Word through music that was fresh, compelling, and adorned with her soft Texas accent.

The album was titled *The Blood+The Breath*, with a subtitle that said it all: *Songs that Tell the Story of Redemption*. In just twelve songs, Caroline painted the blood-red arc of the Bible's Big Story from Genesis to Revelation, and I was amazed how in a few lines she was able to etch cameos of key Bible stories while hewing closely to the Book's great Gospel theme. And Caroline—joined in turn by Abraham, Isaac, Moses, and

Isaiah—pointed me to Christ, the Center of the Story. I'll never forget reaching Jerusalem, the place of Jesus's suffering, sacrifice, and resurrection, with the lines of living hope from 1 Corinthians 15 resounding in my heart when Caroline sang:

> Wake up, wake up
> And listen for the trumpet sound
> For a dead man rose up from the ground
> Rise up, rise up
> You dry bones in the dirt
> For the Son of God has risen up first . . .
>
> Sown in weakness, raised in power
> Sown in dust, death and dishonor
> Raised immortal, never again to die
> Death is swallowed up by life.[2]

I would come to know the singer behind the songs that so strengthened my heart back then, as I met Caroline on several occasions over coffee and at concerts. I also was able to meet her husband, Nick, and their three children. Her love for Christ is boundless, and her music flows from that deep spring. She wrote a song that she calls her "mission statement," and I think one of the stanzas of "Tell That Story" perfectly sums up Caroline's life and music:

> I'm a steward of the Story
> As the moon reflects the light
> So if you see Him and forget me
> I've told this Story right.[3]

Caroline's hands are always full as a wife, mother, neighbor, disciple-maker, songwriter, and musician. When I heard she was working on a new album based on the Psalms, I wanted to see how she juggled her life to do it—and I wanted to hear the music in the making. So I went to Dallas and spent a day with her.

**Dallas, Texas**
**September 20, 2022**

I set out in the morning for Nick and Caroline's place, which was just a short walk from where I was staying. Despite the early hour, the air already hinted of the heat ahead. Texans say that there are twelve seasons in Texas—and most of them have to do with how hot it is. There's Summer, then Hell's Front Porch, with a brief False Fall, followed by Second Summer. Although technically it was Second Summer, it felt more like Hell's Front Porch.

When I reached Nick and Caroline's home, breakfast was underway, and Nick was reading a Scripture passage, as is their habit in starting the day as a family. The day's reading was from Exodus about the call of Moses to deliver God's people from Egypt. Caroline summarized the passage for Ellie, Harrison, and Libby: "Moses said, 'Lord, I can't do this alone.' And God answered, 'You won't have to.'" It was a good reminder for me, too, as I set out to write the story of this day.

Before heading off to school, Harrison brought out his pet lizard—a bristling bearded dragon named Finn—and little Libby brought out an armful of a cat named Oreo. After I met the extended family of pets, they gathered their lunches, books, and backpacks, and we all set out for school. Nick and Caroline walk the two youngest to school, which is conveniently just a block away, and then Ellie walks a bit farther to her middle school. There were lots of greetings of neighbors and kids and crosswalk guards all along the way. I can tell they really know their neighbors—and not just their names. It's obvious they've taken the time to learn their stories, too.

Afterwards, Nick went on to his office, and Caroline and I headed to her "office," a favorite coffee shop in Dallas not far from the studio where she would record some of her Psalms album that afternoon. Morning rush hour was over, and we sailed along the ribbons of asphalt that unwind toward the shiny high-rise horizon of the Dallas cityscape.

Along the way, we passed Elm Street, the site of the assassination of President Kennedy. Seeing the place up close for the first time evoked one of my earliest memories. When I was five years old, I found my mother crying in front of our television set as the shocking news first broke from Dallas. A white X in the middle of Elm marks the place where the fatal shot struck JFK; the street still has the look of a crime scene with the X on the asphalt and the sniper's nest in plain view. It is a brutal, mournful spot—one that is forever stained in my memory by my mother's tears.

We drove on to Caroline's favorite coffee shop, Davis Street Espresso. It's clearly a good place to create and caffeinate. Over strong cortados, she prepared for the day's recording session. We looked over lyrics and talked over a few wording changes she was playing with. The album's still a work in progress, but the chosen psalms touch a range of themes. She told me,

> I'm drawn to the Psalms the same way everyone is drawn to the Psalms—because they run the gamut of emotion. For example, there's Psalm 92, which says, "It's good to give thanks to the Lord!" The song my co-writer, Wendell Kimbrough, and I wrote for this psalm is really upbeat and talks about playing instruments, clapping our hands, stomping our feet, and singing out loud in thanksgiving. But just ten psalms later, you find Psalm 102, which talks of how tears are my drink, I eat ashes instead of bread, I can't sleep or eat, and I plead to God not to hide His face from me. Both Psalm 92 and Psalm 102 are found in the same ancient songbook. We all feel this full range of emotions, and somehow we can pray both kinds of prayers—and everything in between—in the same lifetime . . . and sometimes within the same day. The Psalms can give us words when we don't have words.

I love how these songs have such simple beginnings—whether from a prayer framed by a psalm or scribbled out when a song suddenly writes itself in her heart. Caroline starts the painting with words, and then adds the brushstrokes of voice, rhythm, and instruments. The Psalms album is just part of Caroline's desire to write the stories from the Big Story and put them to music. She said,

> We have a lot of songs out there on the radio about our personal experience with God, and we have a lot of worship songs that talk about the same four or five themes over and over again. I want to write songs about the prophet Nahum and about Isaiah. I like to tell those kinds of stories because biblical literacy and understanding the whole Story of Scripture is something the Church is losing. I want to write songs that help people experience God's beautiful Big Story. Of course, we need the songs about Jesus being with us when we're stressed, but that's only one aspect of His fully orbed character. And we need to be reminded that our place in the Story is not the center.

Our coffee cups had long been empty, and the clock pressed us to move on. We got a grab-and-go lunch at a taqueria and headed over to Paul Demer's recording studio. Caroline hoped to make good progress on recording her Psalm 63 song before heading back for school pickup. Along the way, Caroline played the scratch track (the preliminary recording) of her Psalm 91 song. This has been a psalm I have leaned into throughout my cancer journey, and so I asked her how she came to write the song based on this psalm. Caroline said it was born out of the pandemic by friends who were praying this passage:

> Because you have made the LORD your dwelling place—
>    the Most High, who is my refuge—
> no evil shall be allowed to befall you,
>    no plague come near your tent.

Psalm 91:9–10

I asked her how she balanced the seeming dilemma between praying that passage back to God and seeing that God does not always keep us safe from physical suffering, persecution, or death. She said,

> This is a commonly misunderstood psalm, and I wanted to be careful when writing this song. I looked at commentaries. I listened to sermons. Instead of saying, "I know you'll keep me safe in this life," I tried to write a song that said, "I know you've got me in this life, and you are holding me." Safety can mean physical safety or it can mean the safety of being held in God's sovereign hand. I tried to focus on the latter aspect of safety. After all, God doesn't necessarily promise us physical safety—although He can provide us with that, and it's okay to pray for that. But He certainly promises us the safety of being held in His hand, if we are in Christ.

Her voice was sweet and strong, and her words drew from this favorite psalm of mine.

> My refuge and my fortress strong
> My God in whom I trust
> With you Most High, I make my home
> I shelter in your love
> You keep me like a mother bird
> Beneath your gentle wing
> You guard me as a shield in war
> Your arms protecting me.
>
> But God there is so much to fear
> A threat on every side
> The hunter's trap, the deadly plague
> The terror in the night
> But even if a thousand fall
> I'm held within your hand
> Oh let your angels bear me up
> And strengthen me to stand.

> I'm holding fast to you in love
> I'm calling on your name
> Until at last you raise me up
> To everlasting Day.[4]

I was so touched by these truths again that I asked Caroline to sing this at my funeral. She smiled and told me not to rush things. . . .

We arrived at Paul's studio, a room in his house fitted out for his craft as a producer and a musician. A mandolin and a dozen guitars line the walls—each one is a slightly different "paintbrush" for the fine art of making music. Paul played along on guitar to work through a few ideas with Caroline, but mostly he recorded her vocal track for the Psalm 63 song to which back-up vocals and instruments (whether guitar, keyboard, trumpet, or kick-drum) could be mixed in later. I got a good glimpse of the creative choices that shape and adorn the music that makes an album. Caroline's Psalm 63 had not yet been recorded, so I got to hear the "sweet psalmist of Texas" and the "sweet psalmist of Israel" join together for the first time. Caroline's chorus summarized David's psalm—and so much of her life, too:

> Because your steadfast love
> Is better than life
> I'll open my lips now to praise you.[5]

Afterwards, Caroline and Paul talked through the plans for the next day's recording session, and then it was time to leave to pick up the kids at school. It was interesting to see how she balances the different demands on her. She gets a lot done without seeming to be in a hurry, but Caroline said it hasn't always been this way. She used to think of life's demands like a big boulder she was pushing up a mountain—there was always more work and pushing to do, and if she dared stop pushing, the boulder might

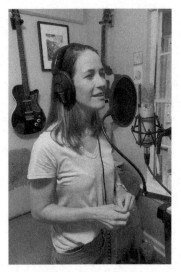

Caroline singing the Psalms

roll back and crush her. But gradually the Lord helped her take her hands off the boulder, so to speak, and filled them with seeds instead, as Caroline saw in the Bible that farming is the better metaphor for the Lord's servants.

Life is filled with hard work, of course, just as it is for any good farmer who expects a harvest. Farmers must plow and sow and weed and, at times, let the soil lay fallow. But at the end of the day, the harvest—big or small— depends on whether the sun shines or doesn't, whether there's a freeze or a drought. It's not all in the farmer's control, and so it is for us. Caroline said,

> In God's Kingdom, success is about being faithful with what we have. Our job is to take the little pile of seeds God has given us and plant them in the little plot of land that God has put in front of us to cultivate. Then we trust Him to let them take root and bear harvest—sometimes a harvest we never get to see.

I asked Caroline how she keeps this faithful farmer's perspective when her life is tugged at from so many sides. She said,

> Gloria Furman told me one time, "God's not schizophrenic. He doesn't have two plans for your life that you're supposed to somehow put together, even though they are incompatible. He's built you to love to write songs, but He's also put you in the place and with the limits and roles that you have here. And somehow those do fit together." I want to tell God's Story through music, but I feel like I can also tell God's Story through

my life at home with my kids, at our school or at our church, by teaching at a Bible study, and by serving on the worship team. In all of these ways I can tell God's Big Story.

Caroline acknowledged the tensions, though.

I could travel more and play more concerts, but in this season I feel like I need to be more present at home. However, that costs me on the music front. I could go to all the conferences and network with all these great people that I love and try to be really present in that world, but I can't because I want to be really present when the kids get home from school. God's called me to both things, and I have to trust Him in the limitations and roles He has given me. It might mean my musical plot of land is smaller, but I know sowing seeds into my three children's lives is also going to reap a harvest.

As we eased off the highway and Caroline navigated the afternoon traffic home, the scratch track for her Psalm 119 song was playing. Caroline summarized the longest psalm into a single song and the chorus into a single sentence, and it's a window into her heart.

I love your word
Because I love you, Lord.[6]

Caroline once told me, "The Bible is the best story ever written, and it's got the best news I know." Being with Caroline and hearing her sing the Psalms that day helped me lift my eyes off myself—off cancer and fear and fatigue—to see our one and only Savior and glimpse the scars in His hands. So in my heart I'm taking up a song, too—one Caroline taught me.

You keep me like a mother bird
Beneath your gentle wing

You guard me as a shield in war
Your arms protecting me.

I'm holding fast to you in love
I'm calling on your name
Until at last you raise me up
To everlasting Day.[7]

# FIVE WITNESSES

Why do I need the word of anyone but God Himself?
He has told me again and again and again that He is
with me and will always be with me, in the deep river,
the hot fire, the Valley of the Shadow. Yet I sometimes
doubt Him. So, in His mercy, He brings along witness
after witness, people who have learned dimensions of
transforming grace impossible for them to have learned
anywhere but where they were.[1]

—Elisabeth Elliot, *A Path Through Suffering*

O f all the memorable mornings of my life, watching the
sun rise on the Sea of Galilee is at the top of the list. I remember how I sat in the dark-to-dawn hour on the north shore
of that storied lake where once Jesus made breakfast for His
disciples. Where they ate good bread and fresh fish together, I
munched on a granola bar and enjoyed a travel mug of coffee;
and as the waves lapped at my feet and the sky brightened, I
thought of all that unfolded there at just such an hour long,
long ago.

Empty-handed and exhausted, the fishermen had nothing to
show for their night-long labor except growling stomachs and
aching arms. As they turned back, the weary disciples bent to

their oars, which glistened as the eastern sky awakened. One of them, John, would never forget what happened next. He wrote that "just as day was breaking" (John 21:4), a stranger called out from the shore and confidently told them if they cast their nets on the right side of the boat, they would find fish. Perhaps with a bit of muttering under their breath and for a chance to prove the stranger wrong, they flung their nets out yet again—and were nearly pulled overboard by the weight of the fish they had snared! As their arms strained to retrieve the full weight of their catch, John likely remembered that three years earlier, this very same thing happened when Jesus first called him, his brother James, and their friend Peter to be His disciples. This was no stranger standing on the shore—"It is the Lord!" (v. 7). John gasped with joy.

That morning, as they sat along the shore and ate breakfast, they talked about what lay ahead. John wrote that this was the third time that Jesus had appeared to His disciples since His resurrection. Despite having seen Christ alive—risen from the dead—they were still uncertain and confused about what it meant. All their plans and dreams had been crushed when Jesus was crucified. Now He was alive, but what was next? What would He do? And what were they to do? Into their confusion, doubts, and fears, the risen Christ spoke with the command of the One who had conquered death. He spoke with the voice of a King whose authority extended across heaven and earth.

He said to them, "This is what I told you while I was still with you: Everything must be fulfilled that is written about me in the Law of Moses, the Prophets and

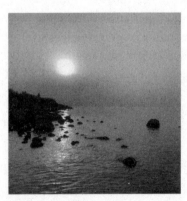

The Sea of Galilee at dawn

the Psalms." . . . "The Messiah will suffer and rise from the dead on the third day, and repentance for the forgiveness of sins will be preached in his name to all nations, beginning at Jerusalem."

Luke 24:44, 46–47 NIV

I can understand these disciples. Twice already they had seen Christ alive—risen from the dead! Yet there they were fishing. The reality of Jesus's resurrection had not yet gripped them, and how His life was to shape the rest of theirs was not yet clear. Perhaps their vision was dimmed by fear and shame, for every one of them knew they had walked away from their beloved friend in His hour of greatest need. Too often we find ourselves as unfocused and unsure as they were. We believe in the resurrection of Jesus mostly as a past truth and a future hope, but it's not a gripping reality in our day-to-day. Because I need reminding, I often repeat to myself the lines of Philippians 3:10 set to song:

> I want to know Christ and the power of His rising,
> Share in His sacrifice, conform to His death,
> As I pour out my life to be filled with His Spirit,
> Joy follows suffering, and life follows death.[2]

Over the years and all over the world I've met believers whose lives bear fresh testimony to the resurrection. They have been strong and necessary reminders to me that even in times of sorrow and suffering, our risen King keeps the last promise He made to us: "I am with you always" (Matthew 28:20). Always. By the time Jesus made this promise, He had already crushed the power of death, so His promise is good on both sides of the grave. "Neither death nor life . . . will be able to separate us from the love of God in Christ Jesus our Lord" (Romans 8:38–39).

The resurrection is more than a fact of history and more than the anchor of ancient creeds. It is our life. *He is risen* are the three words that change everything—and not only on a grand scale but also in the hope that rests over every one of our days until our faith becomes sight.

Here are the testimonies of five witnesses who have shown me truths about this ever-present reality that "He is risen, indeed!"

### Sayid's Testimony: Because Christ is risen, He gives death-defying hope

This brave pastor comes from a Berber tribe in the Atlas Mountains of Morocco. In his 99-percent-Muslim country, he had never met a Christian or seen a Bible. One day while channel-surfing, he came across a Christian broadcast on satellite TV. He was struck by the contrast between Christian prayers for God's blessing on all people and the imam's prayers in his mosque for Allah to curse all non-Muslims.

Through an online contact, Sayid got a Bible and eventually attended a house church. The Christians were patient in answering his many questions, which was a stark contrast to his experience of being slapped in the face for asking questions about Islam. Despite that, becoming a Christian was no easy decision because he knew that following Christ could cost him everything, including his life. But Sayid came to believe on the Lord Jesus and was radically converted. On the day Sayid was baptized, he sent out a group text to all of his phone contacts. It simply said, "Walit masihi" ("I am a Christian"). In his country, this was like asking to be killed, but Sayid did not have a death wish—instead, he has a living Hope.

Sayid now pastors a house church and leads a radio broadcast that is sharing Good News throughout the region. Sayid went to jail for his Gospel ministry and has received many death threats. When I've asked Sayid about that, he has just shrugged off all the hate and intimidation. Because of the resurrection, it's really hard to threaten a man who will live forever.

## Cheryl's Testimony: Because Christ is risen, He stands with His people so they can lean upon Him

I saw this witness to the resurrection in Cheryl Beckett's life. Cheryl served Christ in Afghanistan. For six years she lived in a war zone in a country where death was the official penalty for becoming a Christian—and if the government didn't kill you, family and friends were more than eager to do it.

There is an Afghan proverb that's no joke—it's the plight of millions of women in Afghanistan: "Women belong in the house or in the grave."[3] Cheryl went to the women behind the veil. She learned their language well and served them and their children through health and nutrition programs. She helped them plant gardens and orchards, bringing food and beauty out of that hard land. Her love was legendary. In Gospel terms and using a gardening analogy, Cheryl would always say she wasn't sowing seeds so much as just chucking rocks so others could follow behind her and reap the harvest.

The last time I was with Cheryl, the pressures on the little band of Christians were mounting. Workers had been killed and others forced to flee. I could hear the weariness in her voice, and I was worried about her and her friends. Two months later, while on a mission of mercy, she and her teammates were killed by the Taliban.

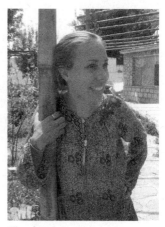

After her death, a friend in Kabul sent me a recording of Cheryl playing guitar and singing lines she had composed from the promises of Isaiah 43. Standing in a rising tide of pressures, perhaps even sensing her own homegoing, Cheryl sang for an audience of one.

Cheryl Beckett

The waters came today, the rivers ran deep.
I saw the waves today; I watched them crashin' over me.
I was drownin' in despair, and I couldn't get up for air.
Then I heard Your voice callin' out to me:

Fear not! I have redeemed you.
Fear not! For I have summoned you by name.
I'm takin' you by the hand, I've placed your feet upon
    dry land,
I will be with you, You will not be swept away.

I felt the burn today, saw the flames beneath my feet,
Walkin' through the fire today, I can't take this heat.
I am drownin' in despair and can't get up for air—
Then I hear Your voice callin' out to me:

Fear not! I have redeemed you.
Fear not! For I have summoned you by name.
You are precious in my sight, so don't give up this
    fight.[4]

"I have summoned you by name." Indeed He has. Even now
I can hear Cheryl singing those words, and I hear in her voice
the fellowship of His sufferings and the power of His rising.

### Wang's Testimony: Because Christ is risen, He saves all who come to Him, including the least likely

Wang was the first Chinese pastor to welcome me to his great
country. By arrangement and to keep a low profile, I was staying in a shabby hotel that was both off the beaten path and
officially off limits to foreigners. However, the owner cared less
for the finer points of the law than he did for paying customers.
Wang and several other Chinese Christians from a network of
underground churches had a vision for reaching the campuses
of their city, and those days we had together of planning and
praying would bring forth fruit that remains to the present day.

The years of our Gospel partnership have not been easy, as the Communists have taken a harder line against Christians. I was in Wang's city the day I learned he and his wife, Jin, had been arrested and their apartment raided. After they were interrogated and had their laptops and Christian literature confiscated, they were released. Wang seemed unfazed and told me, "As a pastor, I always expect to be arrested."

Recently I asked Wang to share his story of grace. It was a beautiful witness of sovereign love and of the reach of the Gospel of the risen Christ!

I grew up in a family that worshiped idols and was involved with all kinds of superstitious stuff, and I started to worship idols when I was young. Though our family hoped to have peace and joy through worshiping idols, it totally failed. My childhood was in such darkness. My tender heart was broken by my parents' quarrels and fights, and I decided not to marry anyone when I grew up. I had no hope for marriage and did not know the meaning of my life.

In 1995, God sent a family from America to my college. I was attracted by the love that Frank and Selina had for each other and their children, but it was their life testimony that attracted me most and drew me near to them. They spent a whole year sharing the Gospel with me in Christlike patience. I gave them a lot of trouble by my questioning. In the beginning, I was against all that they shared from the Bible. Later, even though I could agree on what the Bible says, I still could not believe in God and experienced severe struggling in my heart. I felt I was almost torn into pieces. One evening, I told God if He would not help me, I could not believe in Him. Then God showed HIS great mercy upon me on the very night after I prayed. HE talked to my heart by reminding me of my miserable life from childhood to the present. HE helped me to understand HE is the one who controls my life and cares for me. Meanwhile, the Holy Spirit used the fact of the resurrection of Jesus to help me acknowledge that Jesus is the Son of God. God used the power of the resurrection to overcome my struggling and convince my heart and reason to surrender myself to God. I converted to Jesus in May 1996.

After I became a Christian, I committed to a local Chinese fellowship, which is now the House Church where I have been serving for over twenty years. I experienced amazing healing in my heart through the good marriage example of Mr. Frank. Jin and I got married in 2000, and we have been blessed with a son.

God took an idol worshiper whose home and heart were broken, and pierced Wang's deep darkness with the light of the Gospel. Over the years, "through many dangers, toils, and snares," God continues to grow and use His servant Wang for His glory and fame. Because of the resurrection, the light continues to shine "and the darkness has not overcome it" (John 1:5).

### Gulzar's Testimony: Because Christ is risen, He is preparing a place for His people

I first met Gulzar at the entrance of his church in a town near Lahore, Pakistan. Other members of the Salvation Army church had gathered there as well to sift through the ashes and charred remnants of their church building. Two days earlier, a Muslim mob—with the encouragement of the imam and the complicity of the police—attacked the Christians in Gulzar's town, where the three hundred Christian families are a small, vulnerable minority living like lambs among wolves. All five churches were burned, and many Christians' homes were looted and wrecked. Where they would go and how they would live was anyone's guess. They certainly were not welcome there.

Gulzar stood at the gate of his church, whose door and windows were now just gaping black wounds—and *he* offered *me* comfort. In his broken English, Gulzar told me two promises help him face the fear and loss. He quoted from John 14:1–3, "Let not your hearts be troubled. . . . In my Father's house are many rooms. If it were not so, would I have told you that I go to prepare a place for you? And if I go and prepare a place for you, I will come again and will take you to myself, that where I am you may be also." Gulzar rehearsed our Lord's words with joy—and in the most incongruous setting imaginable. And yet it was, in fact, the perfect promise for outcasts like him. I fully witnessed what was said of first-century Christians: "You joyfully accepted the plundering of your property, since you knew that you yourselves had a better possession and an abiding one" (Hebrews 10:34). And then, quoting our risen Lord, Gulzar added, "Be faithful unto death, and I will give you the crown of life" (Revelation 2:10).

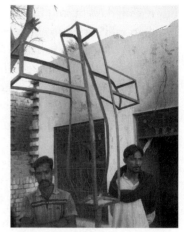
After the attack

### Pavlo's Testimony: Because Christ is risen, He is an unfailing Refuge when our world has been shaken

Russia's war on Ukraine caught my friend Pavlo and his family in the line of fire. Here's the journal entry I wrote about our first contact after many agonizing days of waiting to hear if they were okay. I was surprised that his message was full of joy—joy drawn from the promises of the Psalms and from the presence and help of Jesus during the worst days of Pavlo's life.

*March 17, 2022*
*Artillery Road*

Pavlo was finally able to get a message out to me today. It's been three weeks since the Russian invasion of Ukraine, and within days he and his family found themselves behind enemy lines and cut off from their home and the church Pavlo pastors in Kyiv. As tanks rolled in and power was cut, eventually their cell phones died and communication stopped. But today I finally heard from Pavlo, and he filled me in on their surprising deliverance and all the ways in which the Lord had brightened the dark days leading up to their escape.

Pavlo is a deep student of the Word and a faithful preacher, but he told me he had "rediscovered" the Psalms since the invasion. From the first day of the war, he and his family read aloud from the Psalms and found words of hope and fresh courage. The Spirit-inspired psalms read from his well-worn Bible gave such spontaneous joy that it was as if they were reading them for the first time.

After nearly two weeks without power and with Russian soldiers now looting stores in town, Pavlo and his family decided to set out for the twenty-five-mile walk back to Kyiv. However, Russian troops stopped them, and an officer asked them where they were going.

"Kyiv," Pavlo replied.

"Too dangerous—you will never make it. Turn north and go to Belarus, and you will be taken care of there," the officer said.

Pavlo said the officer was not a convincing liar, so they waited in the road, and eventually the Russians let them pass. Then, remarkably, a school bus came along, picking up refugees, and took them as far as the Dnieper River, where the bridge had been blown up. That day the river was partially frozen, so they crossed on the ice and—over deeper parts—on a tenuous footbridge that had been rigged along the ruins of the bombed bridge. From Kyiv, they had access to highways they could take to the relative safety of western Ukraine or western Europe. But Pavlo had a flock to shepherd in Kyiv, and there were Gospel opportunities during the darkest and most dangerous time that any of them had ever experienced. And so, framed in those terms, Pavlo said the decision was fairly easy—they would stay in Ukraine and serve. That day he and Inna were headed out to visit church members in the hospital and then deliver relief supplies to the needy. Pavlo said there was no fighting in and around the city that day, and the only danger in Kyiv was Russian missiles and bombs!

I could tell he was glad to be back in action and serving. The daily dose of Psalms was still cheering his heart, and he left me with this promise: "But you, O LORD, are a shield about me, my glory, and the lifter of my head. I cried aloud to the LORD, and he answered me from his holy hill. I lay down and slept; I woke again, for the LORD sustained me" (Psalm 3:3–5).

It is fitting that Pavlo should read the Psalms with fresh eyes, for many of them were written from hiding places, on battlefields, or during tear-stained nights by people who knew they would never make it without a Deliverer. The walls of their world were falling apart—they needed a safe place—so the psalmist wrote:

> God is our refuge and strength, a very present help in trouble.
> Therefore we will not fear though the earth gives way, though the mountains be moved into the heart of the sea,
> though its waters roar and foam, though the mountains tremble at its swelling. . . .
> The LORD of hosts is with us; the God of Jacob is our fortress.
>
> Psalm 46:1–3, 11

The walls of *this* refuge are not of stone or steel. These fortress walls are of a more enduring substance, for *God* is the refuge.

———

In my own battle much closer to home, I am learning more of my need to lean on the walls of *this* Refuge. Like the disciples by Galilee, I am still coming to grips with all that the resurrection means for me. The crucifixion shook their plans and expectations, and then their own unbelief and fear shook their relationship with Jesus. Cancer has shaken my plans and expectations. It has exposed my unbelief and given fear a footing. Every refuge I count on that isn't the refuge of God turns out to have flimsy walls and gives only momentary relief. I am reminded that when David was surrounded by enemies determined to kill him, he steadied himself with the greater realities that also surrounded him.

I will sing of your **strength**; I will sing aloud of your **steadfast love** in the morning. For you have been to me a **fortress** and a refuge in the day of my distress. O my **Strength**, I will sing praises to you, for you, O God, are my **fortress**, the God who shows me **steadfast love**.

Psalm 59:16–17, emphasis added

The love and strength of my risen King surround me like a great keep. Like the disciples, in moments of pain or confusion, I often forget the One who promised, "I will never leave you nor forsake you" (Hebrews 13:5). But His patience and cross-centered love steady me when the walls of my world are shaken. "I was pushed hard, so that I was falling, but the LORD helped me. The LORD is my strength and my song; he has become my salvation" (Psalm 118:13–14).

# TOWARD EVENING

For now we see through a glass, darkly; but then face to face: now I know in part; but then shall I know even as also I am known.

—1 Corinthians 13:12 KJV

# ANOTHER WAY TO DIE

In every trial and loss
My hope is in the cross
Where your compassions never fail.
So more than watchmen for the morning
I will wait for You, my God.[1]

—Bob Kauflin, "Out of the Depths"

More than once I've had so close an encounter with death that I've felt the thinness of the wall between this world and the next. Those moments on the edge of my mortality—whether underwater or in a war zone—were at first breathtaking with suddenness and then sobering with realities and what-ifs; but I was too busy living to think much about dying, and soon those close calls were in the rearview mirror.

However, my latest death threat is no near-miss, nor can I outrun it. Twin cancer diagnoses in 2019 and 2021 have struck hard. Unlike my sudden brushes with death, cancer shadows my path every day. But if I can see a kindness from God with this cancer (and I can count many of His kindnesses these past three years), it's that cancer has given me a clearer focus on the finish line—and so I want to make every stride count. In spite of my weakness, I want to finish strong.

I would like to say that I have lived up to the lines on a plaque my mother kept on the kitchen wall for our everyday reading when I was growing up:

> Only one life
> 'Twill soon be passed.
> Only what's done for Christ
> Will last.

But I haven't. The first few months after the diagnosis was a dark time. I wasn't angry or afraid, because I believed my good and sovereign God had brought this—and He does all things well, even if I'm completely at a loss to see it all. But in the weeks after the oncologist said it was stage 4 lymphoma, I was perplexed as to what it all meant. Here is an undated entry in my journal from that time:

> Words come hard. Even as I write this, my journal page is scratched through and nearly illegible. My feelings have been illegible, too, since the day the surgeon said, "It's cancer." I haven't known how to talk about it, and close friends have written to say they don't know what to say. When I told the colonel about the cancer (a man who got me out of a serious situation in Iraq years ago—a soldier and friend I call "The Angel of Baghdad"), he texted back a one-word reply: "Damn." I was deeply touched by the affection in that short, heart-felt expletive. I, too, have been short on words.
>
> My initial reaction to the diagnosis was disgust. Time spent in doctors' offices and hospitals is measured in dog years, and now the prospect of all those appointments, treatments, and waiting room waits is daunting. That's time I had better plans for—time with Debbie and our children. My most painful thought is that my four-year-old grandson won't remember me, that I'll just be a picture in a frame to him. And there are more stories to tell from the remote corners of Christ's Kingdom. I'm ready to fill more pages—to tweak Wesley's words—"O for a

thousand more pages to write of my great Redeemer's praise, the glories of my God and King, the triumphs of His grace."

All these grand plans roll over in my mind as I sit—not in some far country but instead in a waiting room amid its grubby magazines, the TV's mindless chatter, and my fellow detainees here at the cancer hospital. Many of them are so ravaged by cancer and its cures that they snap me out of my self-pity. One of them has the big, calloused hands of a man long accustomed to showing up and doing hard work. Now he was showing up to do the hard work of surviving. Perhaps the conscious, courageous effort to live and die well will be the hardest thing this man will ever do. I saw all of this in his weary, determined face as he brushed past me with his walker when his name was called.

This reminded me of something Spurgeon wrote—words that haunt me in my profound fatigue. "The trumpet still plays the notes of war. You cannot sit down and put the victory wreath on your head. You do not have a crown. You still must wear the helmet and carry the sword. You must watch, pray, and fight. Expect your last battle to be the most difficult, for the enemy's fiercest charge is reserved for the end of the day."[2]

In the months that followed, I received the diagnosis of a second, more aggressive cancer. Cancer will now shadow me until the end, and so I'm navigating this storm, still striving to make my days count.

My situation, though, is no different from what all of us face. Cancer is just another way to die. We all have a certain amount of time, but how much is uncertain. It is freeing to know this if we are living out the truth of Matthew 16:25, where Jesus said, "For whoever would save his life will lose it, but whoever loses his life for my sake will find it." In other words, I can't save—can't keep—my life. I can only spend it. And if by God's grace we spend our days for the glory of Christ, then we will have lived them well, whatever their number.

This is what Moses reminds us of in his majestic Psalm 90. Moses begins in awe of our God, who is not bound by time in any way. The Rock of Ages does not age. "From everlasting to everlasting you are God" (Psalm 90:2). In cosmic contrast, Moses then reminds us to "number our days that we may get a heart of wisdom" (Psalm 90:12). Of course, none of us can add up in advance the number of days we will be given. But what we are to remember is that there *is* a number, although I can't get too concerned about the number of days I have left. Jesus saved me the trouble over that when He said, "Who of you by worrying can add a single hour to your life?" (Luke 12:25 NIV).

I want to spend *this* day well—the one I've been given now. If I'm given another day, another week, another year, another decade—until the number of them is complete—may each of them be gold that reflects the brilliance and worth of God's glory, not the ashes of worthless things, when in that day I stand before the Lord and give an accounting of how I spent all of my days (see 1 Corinthians 3:11–13).

The following chapters are journal entries written in the moment of this ever-changing, yet ever-pressing, battle. Some of the passages are among the most hard-earned sentences I've ever written.

# IN HABAKKUK'S TOWER

It is utterly crucial that in our darkness we affirm the wise, strong hand of God to hold us, even when we have no strength to hold Him.[1]

—John Piper, *When the Darkness Will Not Lift*

**Springwood Cemetery**
**Greenville, South Carolina**
**Sunday, March 21, 2021**

When I was first diagnosed with cancer in 2019, I set a goal for myself to walk or run the equivalent of a marathon each week. For an athlete (which I am not), it wouldn't be much of a challenge, but for me it was a way to push through the fatigue—a hard, stretching goal, but achievable. I was able to keep it up for a while. Just prior to the COVID-19 pandemic, I was in Rome with my son. Fueled by gelatos and cappuccinos and the joy of exploring a mythical city with my son, we walked fourteen miles in one day! In the current phase of this fight, however, I'm doing well if I can get in half a mile a day. These days walking is mostly a way to spend time with Debbie and find some quiet space. That's why old Springwood Cemetery has become our favorite walking trail. Lanes lace its thirty acres, which we usually have to ourselves. And unlike any other place, all of Springwood's ten thousand residents are COVID-free!

The intricate jumble of two hundred years of different monument styles is intriguing—from soaring obelisks to humble fieldstones and from lichen-flecked angels to cast-iron crosses that mark Confederate soldiers' graves. It's a hodgepodge of history, art, mystery, and decay that's as close to ancient ruins as I am likely to find in my city.

This place is unlike modern, more politely named cemeteries—Memorial Parks or Gardens of Remembrance—that are designed along more efficient lines. With their flat, fake granite and faux bronze plaques, they are made for the ease of mowing crews. They're cheap and efficient, and as vapid as a mall parking lot. The epitaphs also must fit the modern form. When I wrote my mother's epitaph, after I wrote her name and dates, I used up my letter allotment with "Beloved Wife and Mother." I couldn't write about how she loved to play the piano or how she taught children's Sunday school for over forty years and pointed so many little ones to Jesus. There wasn't enough room to tell how Mama loved to fish and play baseball or that her eyes were blue-gray, the restless color of mist rising from the sea, eyes she passed along to me along with a lifetime of love. There was no room for any of that on her epitaph.

Our walk through Springwood today turned into more of a wander as Debbie and I read elegies and Scripture chiseled into markers; many of the stones here speak of resurrection hope. There's a peace that has settled over this place and its moss-etched laments—a kind of quiet that only time can bring. This necropolis of Greenville's founding fathers and founding mothers and their children is like the one Wendell Berry wrote of.

In the town's graveyard the oldest plot now frees itself of sorrow, the myrtle of the graves grown wild. The last who knew the faces who had these names are dead, and now the names fade, dumb on the stones, wild as shadows in the grass, clear to the rabbit and the wren. Ungrieved, the town's ancestry fits the earth. They become a meadow, their alien marble grown native as maple.[2]

For some reason, it was one of the littlest graves that stood out to me above the rest. Though nearly a century and a half has swept over this small spot, it does not seem to be entirely drained of its sorrow. In fading letters, it reads:

Our little
Daisy
Daughter of
G. W. & Martha Howard
Born
Feb 2 1876
Died
Oct 8 1877

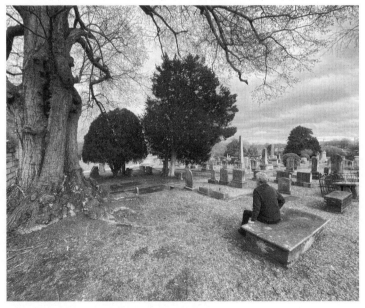

Sitting by Daisy's grave, Springwood Cemetery

Nothing more remains to Daisy's memory. She was only a year old, and the curtain of joy and pain is pulled back in these simple words: "Our little Daisy." The curious thing is that the roots of a great oak have spread to Daisy's grave. The tree would have been only a sapling when Daisy's grieving parents laid her to rest, and it's as if something of Daisy lives on in this ancient oak. Every spring since the sorrow was fresh, the oak's green buds have unfurled to shade this spot. And every autumn, this old tree bends to scatter scarlet leaves on her grave.

Daisy is in the older section of the cemetery on the high ground, near the iron gate. Looking out over the crowded acres, I can easily see a thousand grave plots in a single view. What a small impression we leave behind. But I see no freshly dug graves—there's no more room. Death seems properly gentrified in an old cemetery like this. There is something about those six-foot-deep rectangles with their fill dirt nearby that has always revulsed me. In the South, where the clay is red, an open grave seems even more like a wound in the earth.

I have a thirty-year-old memory etched in my mind from the war in Bosnia. I was in the bombed-out city of Mostar, which was still being shelled by the Serbs, but a shaky truce was holding that day. A city park had been turned into a makeshift cemetery, and the gravediggers, seizing an opportunity to get ahead in their work without having to contend with snipers, were busy with shovels, cutting more ugly scars in the ground, ready to receive tomorrow's inevitable victims. Death the Insatiable ruled that place, just as it does on this quiet hillside. Death seizes all alike, including little Daisy.

I grieve for Daisy, this short-lived flower; but maybe deep down I'm grieving for myself as much as anything, because there are days in my profound weakness when I feel I will not get my full quota of years. Even if I should reach my three score and ten, those years will likely be hollowed out and haunted by cancer. Even now my hours, stalked as they are by nausea or lost in the haze of painkillers, don't seem to count for much. I know it's presumptuous, but I've found myself asking with David, "What profit is there in my death, if I go down to the pit? Will the dust praise you? Will it tell of your faithfulness?" (Psalm 30:9). And I cry with David:

> Be gracious to me, O LORD, for I am languishing;
> heal me, O LORD, for my bones are troubled.
> My soul also is greatly troubled.
> But you, O LORD—how long?
> Turn, O LORD, deliver my life;
> save me for the sake of your steadfast love.
> For in death there is no remembrance of you;
> in Sheol who will give you praise?
>
> Psalm 6:2–5

And again, "He has broken my strength in midcourse; he has shortened my days. 'O my God,' I say, 'take me not away in the midst of my days—you whose years endure throughout all generations!'" (Psalm 102:23–24).

Mine is certainly not a short-lived life like little Daisy's, but there are days in which I feel I'm in Habakkuk's Tower, asking questions and, like him, waiting for answers that don't come:

> I will take my stand at my watchpost
> and station myself on the tower,
> and look out to see what he will say to me,
> and what I will answer concerning my complaint.
>
> Habakkuk 2:1

I'm not yet in Habakkuk chapter 3, where a kind of cancer of promised judgment is about to strike and strip the prophet's world with the force of a relentless army, and yet, where

173

Habakkuk took joy—defiant, triumphant joy—in His Savior, entirely apart from his circumstances:

> Though the fig tree should not blossom,
> nor fruit be on the vines,
> the produce of the olive fail
> and the fields yield no food,
> the flock be cut off from the fold
> and there be no herd in the stalls,
> yet I will rejoice in the LORD;
> I will take joy in the God of my salvation.
>
> Habakkuk 3:17–18

Today, as I rest in the shadow of Daisy's tree, feeling the weight of my weakness, I admit I'm still up in the Tower.

Those who say death is just part of life sound so matter-of-fact, so smug and brave and philosophical—but I think they're just whistling in the dark. Christians have their own versions of this with sugar-sweet songs about suddenly finding ourselves walking around heaven and breathing celestial air. The problem is that it hopscotches right over car wrecks and ventilators and cancer and digging little graves. For believers, "It is not death to die"[3] is only half true. On the farther shore of the last river, where faith becomes sight, the glory and grace of the Lamb is beyond imagining—and He will never forsake His own, even in the crossing of those fearful waters. With Him, life is beautiful, abundant, and forever. *But on this side*, there is still a raging river to cross.

This is how John Bunyan describes the moment Christian and his companion Hopeful come within sight of Heaven's Gate—but between them, they find a barrier that must be breached.

> So I saw in my dream that they went on together till they came within Sight of the Gate.

Now I further saw, that betwixt them and the Gate was a River, but there was no bridge to go over, and the river was very deep. At the sight therefore of this River, the Pilgrims were much astounded, but the men that went with them, said, "You must go through, or you cannot come at the Gate."

The Pilgrims then began to enquire if there was no other Way to the Gate; to which they answered, "Yes, but there hath not any, save two, to wit, Enoch and Elijah, been permitted to tread that path, since the foundation of the World, nor shall until the last Trumpet shall sound." The Pilgrims then (especially Christian) began to despond in his mind, and looked this way and that, but no way could be found by them, by which they might escape the River. . . .

They then addressed themselves to the Water, and entring, Christian began to sink . . . And with a great darkness and horror fell upon Christian, so that he could not see before him.[4]

The pilgrims made it safely to the farther shore, for the King never, ever abandons His own; and He shall also be with me—in and through and beyond the river, but there is no bridge or boat ride across. So while I know that through Jesus "all death can now do to Christians is to make their lives infinitely better,"[5] death is no friend. Death is my enemy, and I hate it. I rage with Dylan Thomas, as he says in his poem "Do not go gentle into that good night; . . . Rage, rage, against the dying of the light."[6]

I rage because death is all wrong. Because we bear the image of our Life-giver, we were made to live, not die. Yet when we turned away from the Giver of Life, our sin brought death in its wake—fearful, inescapable death. I wonder if the full weight of the curse didn't break Adam's and Eve's hearts until Abel's blood cried out from the ground, until they wept over their son's grave, the first grave to tear the earth. Death was terribly wrong—not completely normal. There was no "circle of life"— only a circle of death that the Life-giver alone could break.

And He did!

But to do so, Jesus would first fully experience death. It would mean enduring the tearing of loved ones from Him by Death's claim. Jesus stood at His friend's grave, and even though He knew He would raise Lazarus from the tomb in a matter of moments, Jesus groaned and wept—eyes red, cheeks wet, short of breath, heaving grief.

And it would also mean facing His own death. Gethsemane was no mere midnight prayer meeting. It was a terrible and deeply human crisis. It is heartbreaking to read of His falling to the ground in crushing agony, His face streaked with bloody sweat and tears, while calling repeatedly, "Father, let this cup pass from me!" As the writer of Hebrews says, "In the days of his flesh, Jesus offered up prayers and supplications, with loud cries and tears, to him who was able to save him from death" (Hebrews 5:7).

But Jesus also prayed, "Nevertheless, Thy will be done," and He took and emptied that awful cup and finished what He came to do. As Spurgeon said, "It seemed as if hell were put into his cup; he seized it and at one tremendous draught of love, he drank damnation dry."[7]

Jesus truly understands the suffocating weight of my weakness unto death. Like my Lord, I will be sown in dishonor but raised in glory. I will be sown in weakness but raised in power (see 1 Corinthians 15:43). So I take up my part in the taunt that George Herbert wrote when Christian called out Death:

> Christian: Alas, poor Death, where is thy glory?
> Where is thy famous force, thy ancient sting?
> *Death: Alas poor mortal, void of story,*
> *Go speak and read how I have kill'd thy King.*
> Christian: Poor death! and who was hurt thereby?
> Thy curse being laid on him, makes thee accurst.
> *Death: Let losers talk: yet thou shalt die;*
> *These arms shall crush thee.*

Christian: Spare not, do thy worst.
I shall be one day better than before:
Thou so much worse, that thou shalt be no
more.[8]

Herbert put it powerfully and poetically. Andrew Peterson put it pointedly that Jesus has "beaten Death at Death's own game!"[9] And so, here in the shadow of Daisy's tree, my sympathetic Savior with scarred hands is drawing me down from this tower.

Not with answered questions, but simply with Himself.

# CHEMO DAYS

The way a crow
Shook down on me
The dust of snow
From a hemlock tree

Has given my heart
A change of mood
And saved some part
Of a day I had rued.[1]

—Robert Frost,
"Dust of Snow"

*July 29, 2021*

Debbie and I had the day off. Between errands and getting ready to pack for our long-anticipated beach week at St. Simon's Island, we went to downtown Greer for cappuccino and tea. Afterwards, we walked down Trade Street and looked in the shop windows until we came to the corner next to the old red-brick Davenport. I remembered how we danced outside after our son's wedding here—and today we danced in the street again. As I held Debbie's hand, it felt like the first time—her hand still fits in mine like the last piece of a puzzle.

We got home about noon to start packing. I had said only a category 5 hurricane making landfall on St. Simon's Island would keep us from going on this trip. "Landfall" came at noon, when Dr. Chowdhury called with the diagnosis from the Mayo Clinic: anaplastic large cell lymphoma. It's an extremely rare and very aggressive T-cell lymphoma. She asked to see us right away, so we met with her at four o'clock. She urgently recommended that we not go to St. Simon's next week. Instead, she wanted to aggressively respond to this cancer with chemotherapy.

Afterwards, we called Sarah and Tim and broke the hard news. I hurt that I can't care for Debbie as I should. She lay on the bed sighing and quietly sobbing, and all I could do was hold her as the sun sank red on this day.

### Chemo Day 1
**August 3, 2021**
**Cancer Clinic Infusion Center**

My first chemo day. I've been here for three hours and have another two to go. They are doing the infusions more slowly on this first round—trying to take it easy with the new kid on the block.

The infusion room occupies one whole side of the cancer center. It is reached by a hallway that ends with an ominous door covered with warning signs, as if beyond it lay the core of a nuclear reactor or the Death Star. Until now, I've been able to avoid this place—but that ended today. Today marks a milestone in my cancer journey. Or perhaps, like the entryway, it is more of a warning sign than a mile marker. I will have six of these chemo days with three weeks between each for recovery. Lord willing, everything will stay on schedule so I can finish before Thanksgiving.

Beyond the door, inside the Death Star, it's not so forbidding— basically a large room with a sea of recliners. It's like a La-Z-Boy furniture showroom—except the "customers" are tethered to IV pumps and bags of fluid, and many have lost their hair.

Even though I sit in the company of the condemned, I sense a casual camaraderie. We each face our own fights, but for a few hours we are thrown together in the same recliner-lined arena.

Debbie stayed with me to see that I got settled in, but I encouraged her to take off. No need for both of us to sit here. During her lunch break, Dr. Chowdhury came by—mostly for a pep talk. She is a most remarkable oncologist: caring, competent, and tenacious. If I recounted the thread of providence that led me to her, it would appear tenuous indeed. But I count Dr. Chowdhury as part of God's sovereign, steadfast love toward us in this narrowing valley. So I can say with Solomon of this thread, "A three-fold cord is not quickly broken." Debbie and I feel we have a guide and friend to help us navigate this cancer maze, and at the office visits we talk about more than platelets, hemoglobin, and my hepatic function panel. Because I've traveled throughout her homeland of Bangladesh, we speak of the stories and places we both hold dear. And to cap off an appointment, she has sometimes brought me a plate of good Bengali cooking straight from her kitchen!

Of God's kindnesses today, I have to mention my infusion nurse, Alex. She is attentive, calming, and professional. But from some things she said and advice she gave, I sensed that she knew more about chemo than just the nursing side. Turns out, just two years ago she had her own battle with lymphoma and sat where I am sitting now. Alex experienced the fear, the loss, and the humiliation of cancer. And she also experienced good care. After she came through it, already an RN, she redirected her career path here to help patients at this critical juncture of their journey. I'm sorry for what she has suffered but thankful to have her here today.

Alex kept infusing bag after bag of fluid through the IV pump—drugs ranging from anti-nausea meds to the actual chemotherapy drugs. I could see them go down the drip line into a tube that runs from my arm to my heart. Out of sheer boredom

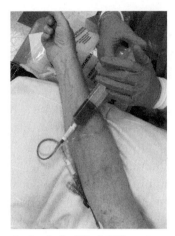

Getting the "red Kool-Aid"

I can watch the drops slowly form up like an Olympic diver preparing for the plunge and then hurtling down the plastic tube. It's incredibly uninteresting, but it's another way to kill time here in the La-Z-Boy showroom.

One of the chemo drugs, though, grabbed my attention. It came in two large syringes to be injected directly rather than through the drip line. The evil-looking vials are marked "HAZARDOUS AGENT—HIGH RISK" and are filled with a sickly red liquid. Alex donned special protective gear and extra gloves to administer this Kool-Aid chemo. While she did that, I crunched on ice chips to help prevent mouth sores. This chemo is a blister agent in the same family as mustard gas. It reminds me that what is delicately referred to as chemo "therapy" is really chemical warfare on cancer cells. I just hope over the next four months the chemo will kill the cancer before it kills me.

There's a nice young chaplain moving around from patient to patient. I keep hearing him say the same thing to each of his recliner-bound parishioners: "Tell me about your feelings." I'm avoiding eye contact and hope he doesn't come by here. I don't feel like talking to him about how I feel. I just want to get off the Death Star.

### Chemo Day 2
### August 24, 2021

My three-hour infusion is nearing its end. I had one ugly, unpronounceable chemical cocktail after another put into me. Some of these drugs would probably kill me if I drank them (especially the red Kool-Aid), but injected into my blood, they may help extend my life. It's weird. I wonder if there will be a future day when chemo treatments like this will be looked at as being as barbaric as leeches are to us today. Probably. Hopefully. But it's where we are now, and it's very much where *I am now*.

To occupy my time, I've been reading and rereading 2 Corinthians 4, especially to better understand that last paragraph.

> So we do not lose heart. Though our outer self is wasting away, our inner self is being renewed day by day. For this light momentary affliction is preparing for us an eternal weight of glory beyond all comparison, as we look not to the things that are seen but to the things that are unseen. For the things that are seen are transient, but the things that are unseen are eternal.
>
> 2 Corinthians 4:16–18

Lord, I believe. Help, thou, my unbelief. Especially on chemo days. Especially on days of uselessness, isolation, and those stabs of fear that come without warning. Help my unbelief.

It's easy to see my outer self wasting away when my strength is gone, my hair is falling out, there's bone pain, my arms are covered with blood blisters, and powerful poisons seep into my veins to kill the cancer that is wasting me away on the inside. So, it's easy to see the wasting away, but it's harder to see the day-by-day renewal.

But the Lord in His patient kindness and good timing has indeed helped me not to lose heart, and to see Him even more clearly beyond these chemo days and their miserable aftermath. Joni Eareckson Tada just sent me a letter. Though she had no idea of this passage I'm struggling with, Joni's timely words struck like a well-aimed arrow:

> I realize this battle against cancer weighs so heavy on your heart. And, Tim, when things are this hard, you know as well as I do that we need the constant renewing grace of Jesus. Otherwise,

we simply lose heart. I recently read this by John Piper: "'Not losing heart' is the discovery of a fountain of life. The refreshing, renewing, strength-giving drink you took in the morning that kept you from losing heart must be taken again the next morning—and night and noon. To 'renew' means that something runs out. The bucket leaks. The car runs out of gas. So, we all need to be renewed daily."

Oh, Tim, I am constantly praying that you do not lose heart. One of my favorite scriptures is 2 Corinthians 4:16–17, "Therefore we do not lose heart. Though outwardly we are wasting away, yet inwardly we are being renewed day by day. For our light and momentary troubles are achieving for us an eternal glory that far outweighs them all." That's us, Tim and Debbie. So be comforted that you are not alone. The Holy Spirit is your champion, and he is constantly "on the call" as you wage war against those renegade cancer cells. We're on your side, the Lord's side. . . .

—Joni

There's iron in her quiet, confident words to not lose heart. Joni has suffered so much in the arena of life as a quadriplegic and with her own battles with cancer. Yet her joy and trust in Christ have magnified Him in stunning ways throughout unimaginable and unimaginably long suffering. Joni is a warrior for Christ. She's shaking me out of my self-pity with its blinders to see the unseen and cheering me on. I can almost hear her saying, "Get out of your foxhole. Look at our brilliant Captain. He's leading the way. Follow closely after Him. Hope and life are in His bright wake!" My fellow soldier has helped me lift up my eyes beyond the drip lines, the blood blisters, and this wasting-away world around me, to catch glimpses of unending glory.

### Chemo Day 3
### September 14, 2021

On one side of the infusion room is a bank of windows. The corner recliner next to the windows is open, so I grab it. Just like on a plane, I always go for the window seat! I'm now settled into my corner office, and the chemo is flowing. Outside there's a coppice of papery river birches, and the trees are filled with birds on this lovely day. I can see goldfinches, cardinals, and sparrows playing in the trees, while cinnamon-sided towhees poke through the fallen leaves looking for lunch. Right now there is more life out in the birch grove than on this side of the window. Everyone's thoughts are their own, and the only sounds that break the silence are the IV pumps that sit and hum the same old tune for us.

The remarkable thing is that I'm not supposed to be here today. Last week my white blood count plummeted to almost zero. Dr. Chowdhury did all she could to keep me out of the hospital because the place is literally overrun with COVID patients, and the stats don't favor my survival if I catch it. She said, "The hospital is not a safe place for you," and gave me her personal cell phone number and said, "Text me day or night if you start to run a fever." And when the fever came, she responded to our text within one minute with instructions of what to do that night—and to see her first thing in the morning. When we did, she made it clear that with my blood count so dangerously low, my next chemo would have to be postponed.

But yesterday morning when I came back for a follow-up visit, my bloodwork numbers revealed that in just three days, my white blood count had moved from nearly zero to normal. We all shook our heads in wonder and thanked God together!

So here I am, chemo day is back on! It's strange that something as miserable as chemo day—especially the sickening side effects—would be a happy occasion. But I'm actually happy to be here because it keeps up the pressure on the cancer—"better living through chemistry," as the old DuPont ad used to say. Right now, if I'm able to stay on schedule, I'll indeed finish chemo just before Thanksgiving—and that will be thanksgiving indeed!

And I'm happy to be here today because there has been such a stirring of prayer that I know God has done this. As Job says, "For he will complete what he appoints for me" (Job 23:14). Lately there have been days that were emptied by weakness, when just getting over the finish line in the evening was a win. And often on those days when darkness was gathering, notes arrived from friends telling us that they were praying—specific, believing prayer. The timing of these was so perfect that it seemed that God Himself was the mail carrier!

These messages aren't just a quick pat on the back. From Asia and Australia and Africa and across America have come many notes saying that believing prayer for us is being offered up by families and in scattered house churches. They are forceful and specific like this one: "Our entire church gathered last night to pray for you." Another recent note said, "My wife prayed that Debbie would feel that she is being carried and that she would know the complete favor of God upon her apart from her performance. And I was thinking of John 15 for you and asking for fruitfulness in a way that can come only from abiding and remaining in Him."

John Piper sent a note saying he was praying specifically not just about white blood counts and fevers but also for a clearer vision of Christ and the glory of His all-conquering love for me:

> I am praying that your vulnerability to infection will be enveloped in the hands of the all-seeing, all-powerful, all-protecting God of grace. "In" all these things we are more than conquerors. "In" a zero blood count, Lord, grant Tim to conquer! Conquer with great faith. Conquer with sweet peace. Conquer with freedom from infection. Conquer with lucid heart-sight of the glory of Christ.

This victory today is but a battle within a war. The outcome of the war, which was secured by my risen King, has never been in question. But the battles in this long campaign turn with the days—and some days are better than others. In all of them, though, I am greatly loved. The songbirds outside the window remind me it is so. For Jesus, in calming the fears of His people, said, "Look at the birds of the air: they neither sow nor reap nor gather into barns, and yet your heavenly Father feeds them. Are you not of more value than they?" (Matthew 6:26).

God is good to let me be here today, and He's good to send the sparrows to keep me company. Inside, our IV pumps hum their tuneless tune, but outside, the birds are singing in the birches. I have a song, too. It's an old hymn that I only recently learned, and it helps me rehearse my hope.

> What tho' my joys and comforts die?
> The Lord my Saviour liveth;
> What tho' the darkness gather round?
> Songs in the night he giveth.
> No storm can shake my inmost calm
> While to that refuge clinging;
> Since Christ is Lord of heaven and earth,
> How can I keep from singing?
>
> I lift my eyes; the cloud grows thin;
> I see the blue above it;
> And day by day this pathway smooths,
> Since first I learned to love it,
> The peace of Christ makes fresh my heart,
> A fountain ever springing;
> All things are mine since I am his—
> How can I keep from singing?[2]

### Chemo Day 4
**October 5, 2021**

Dawn was as dark as night. It's a bleak, wet morning. Thunder rolled like a kettledrum, and a downpour darted in the headlights as Debbie drove me to the cancer center for the first

187

appointment of the day. Not sure how I drew the short straw. When we arrived, I got a quick kiss and then hit a wall of water in the dash to the door. She will return in five hours when chemo is done and I'm too wobbly to drive.

These days when I'm too weak, Debbie is often my driver—as well as my pharmacist, medical navigator, and scheduler—in addition to her usual master juggling skills of managing home life and our work at the mission. For much of our forty-one years of marriage, our life together has meant living apart from each other, but Debbie has always had a remarkable calmness about my restless dreams and risky travel, and has always sent me out backed by her love. She reminds me of astronaut Michael Collins's wife, Pat, who slipped the poem "To a Husband Who Must Seek the Stars" to her husband before he set out for the moon. It included these lines:

> Where is the comfort for my soul?
> You, my love, have helped me know:
>
> I'll be unafraid, undaunted.
> Yes, of course! I need not face
> Any peril; or be haunted
> By the hazards you embrace.
>
> I could have sought by wit or wile
> Your bright dream to dim. And yet
> If I'd swayed you with a smile
> My reward would be regret.
>
> . . .
>
> Take my silence, though intended;
> Fill it with the joy you feel.
> Take my courage, now pretended—
> You, my love, will make it real.[3]

Debbie always sent me on to the ends of the earth with all her love and trust. I remember how she packed my luggage for me (I never even bothered to look inside until I was on the other side of the world), and often she tucked a love note in there, too. Together we shared the same joy and adventure of following Christ. Our hearts were bound together in this as if we were skipping along hand in hand—even when we were separated by an ocean.

My globe-trotting world has become much, much smaller. Some days I'm too weak to cross the street, much less cross a border. Instead of buckled in seven miles up, looking down on Greenland's glaciers or Arabian deserts or the wrinkled face of the Himalayas, I'm in a recliner at the cancer center tethered to an IV pump. I'm frustrated in this smaller world where walls seem to be closing in more and more—walls of my own weakness, walls of isolation because my immune system has been broken by cancer and its cures, walls of lost time. Not just lost in its swift passing but lost to my control as appointments blot my calendar. How many hours—week after week, month after month—are swept away in well-named "waiting rooms" and with doctors and nurses for scans, blood draws, and chemo? Whatever illusion I ever cherished that I am in charge of my time is laughable now.

My world is slower now, too. Cancer has been a hard brake on my sun-chasing days. I remember a time when I caught an early flight out of California bound for New York. I watched the sun rise over the San Jose Mountains and then watched the sun set that day from the Brooklyn Bridge, as last light left the towering cityscape of Manhattan in silhouette like another Stonehenge. The next day I flew to Moscow, then caught a flight to Armenia, and by that evening I was on the plains of Ararat in time to watch the sun set over Noah's country. Motion. I miss it. Life is much slower today as I sit and watch my drip line and the rain spattering the window next to me.

I cannot deny my frustration and restlessness, but my smaller, slower world has helped me open my eyes and see what is in front of me. There are discoveries every day, and the best of these daily discoveries is Debbie. We've spent more extended time together this year than ever before. I've seen the weight of my cancer on her, and not being able to protect her from this has been a hard and humiliating stab to my weakness. Yet all along Debbie has carried my burdens with a steady, sweet—though sometimes tearful—tenacity. I've come to know her better and to love her more, and am mystified at how she could love me so much. Debbie's love for me has been more evidence of God's love for me. Grace upon grace.

How did I get to marry such a woman? I could have written the words John Newton penned to a friend about his beloved Mary. John and Mary had been married for nearly as long as Debbie and I have when he wrote,

> Our setting out in wedded life was something like that of an adventurous mariner, who should put to sea without either pilot or compass. We knew and thought but little of the Lord, but he thought of us, his plan was exceedingly different from that we had formed for ourselves, but it gradually opened upon us, and hitherto he has helped us. What is before us we know not, but he knows it all, and I am enabled in some measure to cast the care upon him.[4]

In another place in that same letter to his friend, Newton wrote,

> And though you must expect to meet with some storms in such a world as this, you have a right to look up to the infallible pilot, whom both winds and seas obey.[5]

That is a good word to remember on this dark, rain-swept morning when all I can do is look up.

### Chemo Day 5
**October 26, 2021**

From my study window the light is long and low, sifting through the west woods—my little backyard stand of oaks and maples with dogwoods just beyond my reach. The dogwoods are nearly stripped, the holdouts hanging on for dear life and dangling in this golden hour like so many bits of stained glass. The sun brightens the cracked leather faces of books on my shelf before settling in among the comfortable clutter of pictures and swords and memories that surround me.

This was supposed to be chemo day 5, but in a surprising twist this weekend, I got a blood clot in my jugular vein that was triggered by the PICC line that runs from my arm to my heart. Further use of the line could cause more blood clots, so the line was pulled out this morning and my infusion postponed until next week. So instead of getting chemo and red Kool-Aid, I got ice cream with Debbie, and we walked downtown under a perfect October sky.

It used to be that on our walks, Debbie would ask me to slow down. Now on our walks, I know that I am slowing her down. Perhaps this is a better pace anyway. My hurry before was for hurry—something between walking and running, whether on streets or on stairs, which I'd always take two steps at a time—*three* was even better! But I missed things along the way, things lost in the blur. Today I saw more. The maples on Main were dressed in fall fashion, and above us the cirrus clouds formed into a flock of seagulls with white wings swept out across a sky so blue it hurt to

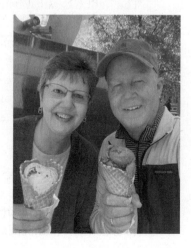

look at it. There was architecture to admire, statues to pose with, a candy store to investigate, and beside me this beautiful woman whose hand, as always, fits in mine like the last piece of a puzzle. I love the warmth of her skin and the taste of her lips. The afternoon hours tripped along and were sweet and so complete that we could almost forget what we were trying to forget.

My oncologist made it clear last week that my chemo treatments were working well in fighting the T-cell lymphoma, but that good news is now paired with the troubling news that this cancer is so aggressive that even with the effectiveness of the chemotherapy, it is likely to be back in less than a year, possibly even just a few months. By then nothing will be able to be done to stop it. However, because the chemo has been effective, I'm a candidate for the only other treatment option left to me—an autologous stem cell transplant. It's a daunting path for us—a real gauntlet—but it is a risk we are willing to take because it holds the prospect of several years of normal life and possibly even a cure, if I can get through it. My last chemo day was to be a finish line—now it's merely a milestone before the path plunges into a narrowing valley.

The light has faded behind the dogwoods. Brilliant leaves that were like the windows of Sainte Chapelle a few minutes ago are dull now and tremble in the growing darkness. In the spring, the arms of these trees will be sleeved in green and offering bouquets of pure white blossoms, but a deep winter must pass between us before April can come and kiss the land with promise. I hope to see that miracle yet again.

*Chemo Day 6*
*November 22, 2021*

Another morning drive to the cancer center. A cold rain swept through last night, stripping many of the trees. It was autumn's first shiver here, and beneath a flannel sky, the sodden maples look like tintypes. There is both beauty and sorrow in their spare lines and the losses of the night. Were there time, I would like nothing better than to walk among them. Robert Frost kept company with his melancholy among such trees, and they draw me, too:

> My Sorrow, when she's here with me,
> Thinks these dark days of autumn rain
> Are beautiful as days can be. . . .
> Not yesterday I learned to know
> The love of Bare November days
> Before the coming of the snow.[6]

Debbie gave me a kiss in the parking lot before heading to the office, and I went to the La-Z-Boy showroom and took a seat. Jack, my nurse today, finally found a good vein and got me hooked up and underway. Sam came by to see me. She's the nurse who gives me a shot in the stomach each time to boost my blood count. Sam is fun and likes to quote Muhammad Ali just before I get the jab: "I float like a butterfly and sting like a bee!" We laugh a lot. But not so much today. She just learned that the stem cell transplant is next for me. Worry seemed to weigh on her assuring words this morning as I prepare to move on.

Yes, moving on, but not like I expected. Today—chemo day 6—was to be the finish line of this nearly four-month-long marathon. Out of the starting blocks last August, I was imagining today would be high fives and celebration and remission and freedom. I guess that's the Walter Mitty in me. With the transplant just ahead, the narrow valley I'm in just closed in further—now down to a single path that leads into a room in the Bone Marrow Transplant Unit. It is the path through the valley of the shadow of death. I do not want to go there, but I will because it's the way forward. But I do not want to.

Psalm 42:10 says,

> As with a deadly wound in my bones,
>     my adversaries taunt me, [my cancer and the Enemy
>     taunt me]
> while they say to me all the day long,
>     "Where is your God?"

On this "bare November day" when, like Frost, "my sorrow" keeps pace with me and the black dog of depression slips his leash, my answers to the taunt feel thin and sound rote. The wound in my bones attempts to sink me, but a rope has been thrown to me, and this morning both the rope and the hands that draw me are strong. I'm gripping the promise earlier in the psalm:

> By day the LORD commands his steadfast love,
>     and at night his song is with me,
> a prayer to the God of my life.
>
>                                 Psalm 42:8

My King's love is all action. The cross is the best proof of that, but with sovereign command He also directs His care for *me* every day and in every way, seen and unseen. It can be as routine as breath and heartbeat but also as surprising as the cherry pie a friend made that arrived yesterday still warm from the oven. God's steadfast love can also cross a dozen time zones because, like my friend Gloria Furman says, "God's mercies are new every morning—and it's always morning somewhere."[7]

I got a message from a stranger on the other side of the world, and his note left me with tears of joy because in it I felt my Father's love. Lawrence "met" me through the *Dispatches from the Front* films that were shown at his church in the Philippines. Somehow, he heard about my cancer and mobilized an army of pray-ers:

*Dear Dr. Keesee,*

*Just want you to know that I and my wife are praying for you daily. We are Filipinos working in Dubai. We will continue to pray for you. There are a lot of us praying for you. Our church here in Dubai prays for you, our church in the Philippines as well. My mom in the Philippines prays for you too.*

*Sincerely,*
*Lawrence and Ethel*

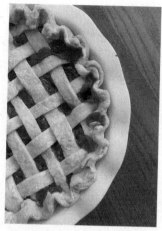

Steadfast love and a cherry pie

So I have seen my Lord's commanding love toward me every day, but there's a part of the psalmist's sentence I still long to hear: "And at night his song is with me" (Psalm 42:8).

My sleepless hours when the medicines have run their course are not peaceful times of moonlit reflection. It's more like a battle, and the fog of war seems deeper in those dark hours. I need to sleep. I need to pray. I need to think through the day ahead—and the days ahead. There is restlessness, confusion, and sometimes stabs of fear.

But the other night, as clearly as if Jesus Himself sang these words over me, the lines of a hymn that I knew in boyhood came back to me with such clarity and peace:

> I hear the Savior say,
> "Thy strength indeed is small,
> Child of weakness, watch and pray,
> Find in Me thine all in all."[8]

# CHRISTMAS DAY

There never had been such a Christmas.[1]

—Laura Ingalls Wilder,
*Little House on the Prairie*

The bootprint of war was stamped on the land. It was 1995, the last year of the fighting in Bosnia, and I was traveling through that shattered country. A shaky ceasefire was holding, and there was hope for peace in the New Year. But now, the bomb-cratered road was as silent as an untimely grave, and all along the way were charred, roofless homes and hollow schools with playgrounds covered with glass and shrapnel, the voices of the children long since swept away by the winds of war. The only sign of life was the grim work of the gravediggers. Then I came to a little town perched on the edge of a river. Night was descending, light snow whirled in the headlights, and there over the blackened, blasted Main Street of the town was a single strand of Christmas lights!

I have never forgotten that string of little lights. It was a sign of hope undaunted by the darkness and death all around. Such defiant hope was good to remember again *this* Christmas.

### Christmas Day, 2021

The house is warm and bright. Supper is done, and the Scrabble board and a tin of Christmas cookies will be brought out soon. But bone pain, nausea, and a crawling restlessness inside have driven me outside for a walk, so I pace the backyard in the dark. High overhead, Orion draws his bow and joins a growing host of shimmering stars. Stars always seem to sparkle more in the winter—perhaps they are shivering in the cold? Beneath this celestial string of Christmas lights, I am down here in the dark. A shadow follows me even on this day—maybe *especially* on *this* day.

I can look up at the stars and see their piercing light, or I can look down and see only shadows. This is surely a day, though, to look up because Christ has come! "The light shines in the darkness, and the darkness has not overcome it" (John 1:5). George Herbert's lines come to mind like the firm hand of a friend to pull me back to realities that are deeper than my pain, more enduring than my fears.

> Awake sad heart, whom sorrow ever drowns;
> Take up thine eyes, which feed on earth;
> Unfold thy forehead gather'd into frowns:
> Thy Saviour comes, and with him mirth:
> Awake, awake;
> And with a thankful heart his comforts take.[2]

I've waited for this Christmas like I have for no other. It's been so long since I've hugged my son and daughter and too long since I've seen my grandson and hatched adventures with him. Since the diagnosis last summer, cancer moved in like an unwanted guest who takes over the house—clearing out the cupboard of stamina and consuming the calendar. I would like nothing better than to evict this intruder with a well-placed kick, but he's attached himself to me—and I live here, too. So my cancer—along with COVID's current reign—have kept us apart. But with the stem cell transplant nearing, I was determined that nothing would keep us from celebrating Christmas together. Who knows how many I have left?

John Piper touched on that in a note to me this morning:

> Noel and I take you to the throne of grace almost every day and ask God to make this stem cell transplant totally successful for stirring up faith and for fitting you for years more of magnifying Jesus with your life. I know that this is a very unusual Christmas for you. Never one like it before. Never one like it again. So I pray you will wring out of it every drop of peculiar grace that your Father planned for you before the ages. We love you.
>
> —John

So we've been wringing the joy out of this day, and my cup is full of its sweetness. Just to be together again to talk and laugh and remember is gift enough, but there were many more gifts—some even wrapped in bright paper. This morning all the lumpy stockings laid out on the hearth and all the presents under the tree waited with the rest of us while I read from Luke 2. My young grandson, Blake, was very attentive—next year he should have the honor of reading the Christmas story for us.

Afterwards, we plunged into the presents, and as quick as you can say "Gloria-in-excelsis-Deo," the stockings were emptied and the gifts given. The floor and everyone's laps were quickly covered in a mix of torn wrapping paper, empty boxes, bags of candy, new books, new clothes, new music, and lots of Legos. I love this Christmas morning chaos with all the surprises and smiles of getting and giving!

Then Debbie made a magnificent brunch, and all around the table we joined hands and prayed and feasted. Later, after our coffee, I played some backyard basketball with Tim until my strength ran out—which wasn't long, but just long enough to get in a few spectacular shots! Sarah took my place, and brother and sister played on. The low winter sun stretched their shadows across their old playground—and across the pages of memory, too. It gave me so much happiness to hear their banter and see their joy in just being together. They played and talked till supper. Those brief sweet hours were a gift of peculiar grace on this Christmas Day.

My special gift to Debbie today was three words inscribed on a board of cherry: **Hope in God**. The words are simple and strong, drawn from Psalms 42 and 43, where three times the psalmist asks the same question and gives the same answer:

> Why are you cast down, O my soul, and why are you in turmoil within me? Hope in God; for I shall again praise him, my salvation and my God.
>
> Psalm 42:5–6, 11; 43:5

The psalmist is talking to himself, preaching to himself. He's where I need to be tonight—where we both need to be, getting hold of our discouragement and downward spiral in the face of sudden change and instead directing our hearts to God, who

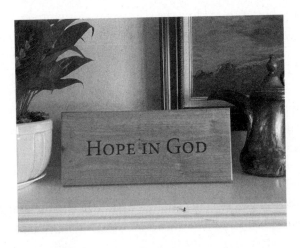

does not change. Our God is a Rock of refuge, and the hope we have in Him is actually hope that He gives—hope rooted in His promises. It's stronger than our darkest days, and it's rooted in the resurrection, so it's stronger even than death.

The plaque will be our reminder as we rehearse our hope in the days ahead—especially the most difficult ones, which will surely come.

The windows glow now in the dark, and our holly tree, which reaches to the roof, is decked in colorful lights—those fat, old-fashioned bulbs that I love to see because they take me back to Christmas nights at my Grandfather Keesee's farmhouse in Virginia. He would always cut down a cedar and string it with big bulbs, tinsel, and tinfoil stars. It fairly took over that little clapboard room where a fine fire crackled nearby. On Christmas night, the house was filled with aunts and uncles and cousins. After supper, my grandfather took out his prized possession: a fiddle that had been his grandfather's, who first played it around campfires of the Confederate Army in a time of war. It was already a century old when my grandfather played it for me, but his strong, worn hands could always draw sweet music from it. On those Christmas nights, he would play and I would sing for all in the house. One of the carols was "O Little Town of Bethlehem." Tonight, the line of "hopes and fears" still rings true and clear, though more than a half century has passed since we made music together.

> Yet in thy dark streets shineth
> The everlasting Light;
> The hopes and fears of all the years
> Are met in thee tonight.

I'm not sure why, but I always liked to go outside and look at the house after supper was done and carols were sung. The old home place has long since been abandoned, but I can still see it in my mind. It was as if the whole day was bound up in that place where my mother and father, my brother and sisters, and my grandparents were gathered, and all the joy we had packed into a few hours spilled out into the night and into my heart. For me it was the last gift of Christmas; the taste of this memory is still achingly sweet. Smoke drifted from the chimney, and there was enough moonlight to follow its trail, while the windows glowed and cast their light out into the cold night. Just like then, the warmth of my own house is now beckoning me away from these shivering stars to wring the last drops out of this good day.

# NUMBERED DAYS

Teach us to number our days.

—Psalm 90:12

Moses's prayer in Psalm 90 is full of breathtaking awe and wonder over the God who is "from everlasting to everlasting" and for whom centuries pass with a snap. He was God before time. He is God who enters time. And He will be God when all our clocks and calendars, histories and monuments are no more. But then, in cosmic contrast, there is another kind of breathtaking awe over just how brief *our* time is. Moses says our lives are "like grass"—here today, gone tomorrow. Even if we are granted a full life with enough birthday candles to set off the smoke alarm, yet with a breath, the fire is extinguished and we soon "fly away." So caught between brevity and eternity, we ask God to "teach us to number our days that we may get a heart of wisdom."

Numbering my days took on additional meaning with the stem cell transplant. The radical procedure began with a countdown that started with six days of "killer chemo" designed to kill every remaining cancer cell in my body. But, since it was unable to separate the wheat from the chaff, the infusions also destroyed my bone marrow function and wiped out my immune system. Every morning I was in the hospital, the nurse would take a marker and write the day's date and the countdown number on a board. Day -6, -5, -4, -3, -2, -1.

Killing the cancer without killing me required the reinfusion—the transplanting—of my healthy stem cells that had been harvested a month earlier. The day of the transplant was Day Zero, and all the subsequent mile markers for monitoring the outcome start at that new beginning, especially the critical first one hundred days after the transplant. So we began the one-hundred-day wait to see if this last weapon against the cancer succeeded in beating it.

The transplant and the tortuous recovery that followed were a battle from the start. COVID plagued my steps from the beginning. First, I got COVID shortly after Christmas, which delayed the transplant. Second, the dramatic uptick in COVID cases triggered a sudden change in the visitor policy so that Debbie was not allowed to visit during my three weeks in the hospital. But she was tenacious, and I got to see her nearly every day when she waved at me from the top of the parking deck on her way to and from the front desk to deliver my daily dose of coffee and freshly baked treats from her kitchen. And one special day I was able to arrange a quick tryst with her when she was making her daily delivery—thanks to the help of a friendly nurse who wheeled me down to the lobby.

Debbie and I also exchanged laundry—and, as usual, I got the better end of the bargain, as she sent clean clothes and I returned dirty ones. Whether it was the basket of freshly folded laundry or the plastic bags of more pungent returns, there were always love notes tucked into the exchange, until sickness overtook me in the days after the transplant and the notes were just one-sided. Of all the hard things I went through—the pain, confusion, zero blood counts, the night I fell twice and had to be restricted, the Hell Week that followed—all my troubles were compounded by not having Debbie there. And I knew not being able to be with me added to her pain, which also added to mine.

There are things we are learning through this experience, but these lessons are not neatly packaged for those who ask, "What is God teaching you through your cancer?" My usual response of "I'm afraid I'm a poor student" is an answer to avoid an answer to a question I don't like. God is certainly increasing our faith, but that is an uneven work, for I am, indeed, a poor student. But thankfully I have a patient Teacher. Yet He's given me no shortcuts or quick solutions. My journey would not make an *Our Daily Bread* devotional, nor fit into a pretty picture on Instagram, and my Teacher has not allowed me to skip to the end. We want to make sense of suffering, but it rarely makes sense. We want the puzzle to come together and look like something meaningful, but too often there are missing pieces.

Elisabeth Elliot, in describing her own suffering, wrote of our tendency to "foreshorten the promises" and to look for a quick, satisfying resolution, but that is not the way of the cross. She said,

> All the Scriptural metaphors about the death of the seed that falls into the ground, about losing one's life, about becoming the least in the kingdom, about the world's passing away— all these go on to something unspeakably better and more glorious. Loss and death are only the preludes to gain and life. It was a temptation to foreshorten the promises, to look for some prompt fulfillment of the loss-gain principle. . . . Faith, prayer, and obedience are our requirements. We are not offered in exchange immunity and exemption from the world's woes. What we are offered has to do with another world altogether.[1]

I know Jesus, the architect and builder of my faith, is doing a work of dismantling and rebuilding in my life. I cannot fully see what He is making, but I sense He is laying out larger windows with grander views of Himself and of what's ahead. Though I am a poor student, I know He loves me and is with me. He's shown me this through all my numbered days, but especially while I was in the hospital when it was too dark to see. In that valley of the shadow of death, there are things that happened that I cannot remember—and there are things I would like to forget. There were also moments so beautiful, so painfully gained, that they run like wine through my mind and color all memory of those precious days.

### Blood and Marrow Transplant Unit
### Day Zero
### January 19, 2022

Today was my stem cell transplant "birthday"—a new beginning for my blood, otherwise known as Rescue Day or Day Zero in the countdown. My immune system and bone marrow function have effectively been erased by the previous six days of

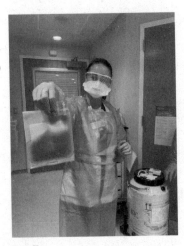

Day Zero

chemo. This morning two nurses brought in a deep-freeze storage device on wheels that looked like R2-D2 (minus the Princess Leia hologram). This unit has held my stem cells at -150°F for the last month. When R2 opened his lid for delivery, the cold, black steam escaped in a cloud, and he looked like he had been hit by a storm trooper!

For all this cutting-edge medi-cine, the transplant process was surprisingly simple. My stem cells looked like cream of tomato soup in a plastic pouch. The nurse put it in a warm bath to thaw, and then the bag was hung on the IV pump and all four million blood cells were returned to me in less than an hour. Everything went well, and afterwards Debbie dropped off a "birthday cake" and a thermos of good coffee to celebrate Day Zero. Now these four million stem cells I got back today need to grow up and flourish over the next couple of weeks.

I don't feel any different, except it's a relief to have cleared this hurdle. Because of the destruction of my bone marrow over the previous six days, I would likely be dead in three weeks without the transplant. In effect, I'm brought to the point of no return, and then I am rescued. All the things that make for life in the blood—red blood cells, white blood cells, platelets—are bound up in these stem cells so that I can have a second chance. As a Christian oncologist told me as he described the transplant, "You have to die before you can live" (see John 12:24).

In a few days, what is affectionately referred to as "Hell Week" will begin. That's when the cumulative effect of all the deadly chemo hits home. I'm told to expect every form of misery, so I'm fighting to be as strong as I can before those days come. Because I now have no immune system, I'm restricted to one place I can walk—a staff hallway the length of a football field. Every night I walk this "Prison Yard." Twenty laps is a mile, and tonight I walked forty. It's hard to know how to prepare for the storm that will soon break, but I know lying in bed waiting isn't the way.

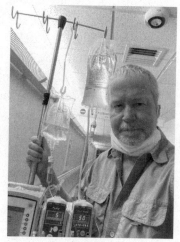

Walking the "Prison Yard"

207

I've been reading passages tonight on God our Rescuer—so many beautiful verses—but I was struck by several passages:

"He rescued me from my strong enemy" (Psalm 18:17).

"For you have delivered my soul from death, yes, my feet from falling, that I may walk before God in the light of life" (Psalm 56:13).

"For he has rescued us from the kingdom of darkness and transferred us into the Kingdom of his dear Son" (Colossians 1:13).

"We felt that we had received the sentence of death. But that was to make us rely not on ourselves but on God who raises the dead" (2 Corinthians 1:9).

What a Rescuer! In the face of the gathering storm, I know this Rescuer holds my days, and they are numbered with care.

### Day 5
#### January 24, 2022

Sometime last night I fell. From the looks of my face, I hit my head on the sink, but all I remember is the nurse finding me on the floor. And then, before she could get help and a wheelchair to take me to X-ray, I got up and fell again.

The X-ray showed only that I have a hard head, which everyone already knows, but now I also have FALL RISK emblazoned on a bright yellow wristband. It might as well be a tattoo for all the hope I have that I will get rid of this restriction before I leave here. This fall is a big setback because I can no longer walk the Prison Yard. I can't even walk around my room without supervision. Weakness and now isolation are overtaking me. I think the hit on my head must be my introduction to Hell Week.

I remembered that a few days ago, Joni Eareckson Tada sent me one of her favorite quotes to encourage me:

"We are journeying; we are moving on, onward and upward; no stop, no stay. Nothing can resist our progress; from night to morning, from morning till night, the one thing in God's universe that moves is His Israel; and every step is a step upward, and every fall is a fall forward."[2]

I can now tell Joni that I've literally tested that last line! From my fifth-floor window, I can see a slice of the western sky wedged between the ICU floor across a courtyard from me and the parking deck where Debbie comes and waves with defiant love. The winter sun is setting in crayon colors and leaves glints of red in the remains of last week's snow. I've been sick in distant places before—in Xinjiang on the far side of China, typhoid in Oaxaca—but tonight just across town from my house, I have never felt further from home.

### Day 7
### January 26, 2022
### From Debbie

The doctor called me this morning and said Tim had a hard night—lots of vomiting and abdominal pain. I wish I could be with him when he feels so miserable and can't do anything for himself. They started him on morphine for pain. They did some tests and ruled out some really bad complications, which was a relief. His labs, while frightening to see, are to be expected at this point in the transplant. Thankfully, he has no fever, and the doctor told me, "Nothing he is experiencing is unusual—it's just unusual that he is suffering so many side effects so quickly and so strongly. Nothing is life-threatening. If it were, I would bring you up to the unit myself to see him." So while I can't be with him, at least I know if things get really bad, they will let me see him.

I asked when he could expect to see any improvement, and she said probably three to five more days, depending on when his counts start to go back up. She also said he probably won't feel much like talking or texting for a few days, so not to worry if I don't hear from him directly, but they will be sure to keep me updated and let me know of any unexpected changes. I am grateful for that.

In the last forty-eight hours, several people have sent me the same verses. I think God knew they were exactly what we needed, and I've been reading and rereading them. In fact, at the end of the last coherent conversation I had with Tim last night, I read these verses to him:

> Fear not, for I am with you;
>> be not dismayed, for I am your God;
> I will strengthen you, I will help you,
>> I will uphold you with my righteous right hand. . . .
> For I, the LORD your God,
>> hold your right hand;
> it is I who say to you, "Fear not,
>> I am the one who helps you."
>
> Isaiah 41:10, 13

Tim and I talked about how personal these verses are: God is with us, and He is holding our right hand. It's a wonderfully comforting thought to me right now that if God is holding my hand and He's holding Tim's hand, we are linked together. (I just wish I could close the circle and hold Tim's hand.) We even shared a laugh about how God's hand must be a whole lot bigger than mine! Together we "rehearsed our hope," as Tim likes to say. We reminded each other that God promises to strengthen and help us. And He tells us we should not fear or lose heart, although honestly, I'm not doing very well with that part today. But I do know we need to experience and trust these promises like we never have before.

**Day 10**
**January 29, 2022**

At four in the morning—*every* morning—a lab tech slips into my room and draws blood. It seems that I never have the same lab tech twice, and some are better at the jab than others. This nightly ritual allows them a couple of hours to get the results before the doctor comes in around dawn to review all the reports and then make rounds.

Getting stuck with a needle for the blood draw from these "vampires" is the worst kind of wake-up call, but last night something beautiful happened. The vampire slipped in at four and turned on a single soft light, which left her in silhouette. I never spoke—I just drew out both arms from beneath my blanket and held them out for her to choose the best vein from among all the bruised ones. She drew blood painlessly, and then—still only a silhouette—my vampire leaned close and whispered, "Keep fighting!"

**Day 14**
**February 2, 2022**

By God's grace, I came home today. Though I am weak as water, I am home. And I am happy. I think of that passage in *Lord of the Rings* when Gandalf breaks the evil spell that binds Théoden: "Breathe the free air again," the wizard says to the king. As Théoden slowly returns to his senses, he says, "Dark have been my dreams of late."[3] Mine too. But today I breathe the free air again.

Debbie made me coffee—only this time she didn't have to drive it across town. I sipped what I could as I sat on my bench in my half-acre woods. The oaks, maples, and hickories were in fine winter form, baring their arms like boxers ready for the ring. I know every one of these trees—some I planted—so it's good to be back among friends!

The fog of war is lifting, and I can think and read a bit better. Debbie had a stack of letters and cards for me to catch up on. So much love has been sent to us. So much believing prayer has been sent up for us. One note from a friend in Georgia put a sword in my hand for the battles ahead. This weapon has grown rusty of late, but now I am ready to wield the weapon of "Remember!" which grows brighter with use:

Tim, thank you so much for the encouraging update of progress, progress that keeps on continuing despite dark times, despite uncertain times, and despite valleys. How great to see a few months into this fight that both your body and your spirit are progressing wonderfully, even victoriously. We will be praying for those requests. Final word—I have been struck recently in Exodus and Deuteronomy when over and over again the Lord counters their well-grounded and rational fears with a single, power weapon: "Remember." May the Lord bless you both in the days ahead not only with clarity looking forward, but also with increased clarity as you "remember" all that God has shown you of Himself in these past years.

—Andy

*Day 45*
*March 5, 2022*

It is a comfortless morning. Murphy died yesterday, and I still feel the weight and warmth of him nestled on my lap, although he is nowhere to be seen. He had been declining for the past three months; the vet said he had lymphoma—how ironic is that? But Murphy bravely kept Debbie company during the long, lonely weeks I was in the hospital. He was so weak when I left that I didn't expect to see him again. Yet Murphy hung on, welcomed me home, and gave me a month of comfort before slipping away.

I never expected to love a cat—or any animal—as much as I loved Murphy. He came into our life at a very important time twelve years ago when our children were getting married and moving away. I can see this only in retrospect, for it wasn't planned that way. We imposed no such expectations on a cat. He came from the animal shelter—a rescue cat—at the urging of our son. I was hesitant, but Murphy quickly won me over.

Whether his name, Murphy, followed him from a previous owner or whether he was rechristened at the pound, I'll never know; but his name seemed to befit that gentle cat—for he was a most well-mannered and amiable companion. The only exception to his impeccable manners was whenever cake or pie were brought out, because Murphy had a serious sweet tooth (several very sharp ones, in fact). He was not above planting a paw in a slice of birthday cake to stake his claim, for Murphy understood that of the rules of cake fights, the only one that counts is that there are no rules!

I polished Murphy's chipped food dish this morning and put it away in a cabinet of my priceless things. Debbie has already packed up his other possessions and sent them away because we cannot bear to see them. He was a great companion in the best of times, and he was a great comfort in these hardest of days. It's a bad time to lose him.

I know that love and loss are inseparable—even love for an orphaned tabby cat—but Murphy's death looms large for me right now. It's more than just the loss of a well-loved pet. His sudden departure is another tearing from my hands and from my heart. His absence is a terribly silent reminder of how fragile my grip is on the people and things I love. Lines I learned from a friend in Afghanistan years ago pound at me this morning as I sit in this emptying place.

> If china, then only the kind
> you wouldn't miss under the movers' shoes or the
>     treads of a tank;
> if a chair, then one that's not too comfortable, or

you'll regret getting up and leaving;
if clothes, then only what will fit in one suitcase;
if books, then those you know by heart;
if plans, then the ones you can give up
when it comes time for the next move,
to another street, another continent or epoch
or world.
Who told you to settle in?
Who told you this or that would last forever?
Didn't anyone ever tell you that you'll never
in the world
feel at home here?⁴

**Day 52**
**March 12, 2022**

"Like cold water to a thirsty soul, so is good news from a far country" (Proverbs 25:25). Unexpected, yet perfectly timed to lift the weight of my weakness, John Piper sent me this good news today:

*Dear Tim,*

*On a bitter cold, but bright and beautiful, Saturday afternoon here in Minneapolis, I am rereading your email and praying and thinking about you and being thankful for your faith. This morning I read this in my Bible reading:*

*"I will sing of your **strength**; I will sing aloud of your **steadfast love** in the morning. For you have been to me a **fortress** and a refuge in the day of my distress. O my **Strength**, I will sing praises to you, for you, O God, are my **fortress**, the God who shows me **steadfast love**" (Psalm 59:16–17).*

*Since he repeats the triad, we can't miss the combination. Strength. Love. Fortress. Which I hear as: God's*

*Strength + God's Love = My Fortress. And Christ secures
the whole because in him there is no condemnation.*

*I pray that you would feel surrounded by and protected
and cared for by the Strength and Love of God. May
he be your Fortress from discouragement and doubt and
fear and pain. And may he fill your fortress with healing
and joy.*

*Affectionately,*
*John*

### Day 72
### April 1, 2022

Discovered the first clutch of bluebird eggs in the backyard. It's
one of the signposts of spring—along with the first crocuses,
snowbells, and daffodils. I whistled a little courtesy call as I
approached the box, and out flew Mrs. Bluebird so swiftly she
startled me. I quickly and carefully took a peek inside, and
there were three little eggs the color of the sky all snug in a nest
of tightly woven pine straw with bits of green grass and a few
blue feathers that lined the basket. I thought of lines learned a
lifetime ago but perfect for today.

> O bluebird, welcome back again,
> Thy azure coat and ruddy vest
> Are hues that April loveth best.[5]

Mrs. Bluebird (now joined by Mr. Bluebird) sat on an oak
branch above me and gave me a good scolding. Even as I slipped
away, they kept up the cussin', which gave me a good laugh.
The reprimand just added to the already raucous bird chorus
that fills our half-acre woods today as my feathered friends find
mates, make nests and babies, and trade stories of the winter
that's past and their plans for the spring. I have plans, too.

**Day 75**
*April 4, 2022*

I got to spend the day with my grandson. My compromised immune system has kept us apart for months, but it was time to test my progress—and it was a gorgeous spring day and adventures were calling us.

Blake and I went to McPherson Park. After poking around the cannons that command the heights at the entrance of this vintage city park, we crossed the creek and raced to the playground. Well, he raced, and I trotted behind, adding enough sound effects so he might think I was gaining on him—but it was never close. My racing days are over.

After a good workout on the play set, we went to the creek and stood on a massive rock that in wetter times makes a waterfall. A copperhead lay sunning himself at the water's edge. Blake was delighted. The copperhead must have been five feet long, and in the shining water, his brilliant-patterned skin shone like liquid snake. We sized each other up, and then he slipped away. Blake's mama need not know about the copperhead.

The day was waning, so we headed back home, where I had a surprise for Blake: a big illustrated biography of George Washington. Before I pulled it out, I said, "Blake, have you ever heard of George Washington?" "No," he replied, "but I have heard of George Washington Carver." Then he quickly proceeded to tell me all the cool things that Carver made out of sweet potatoes. I have to confess that my heart skipped a beat.

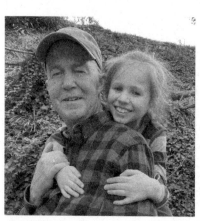

At McPherson Park

What are they teaching kids in first grade? So I said, "Well, let me tell you about who George Washington Carver was named after—George Washington, who is called the father of our country." We read the book together, and I hopefully put a foundation stone or two into his history learning.

After that, we read another book—*What It's Like to Be a Bird*. Every page was an illustration of our God's creative genius in the winged world. We talked about how the birds point us to the God who made them and all that we see.

Whether we're reading or playing, I'm praying—quiet, constant prayer—for my sweet grandson. I've prayed for him since he was a baby, when I would carry him in my arms for hours to calm him and show him things. I keep a picture of us by the last lamp I switch off at night. It's my time and place to pray for Blake. He is growing up in a world of deep deceits and of coercive lies, and I pray that God would bring this precious boy to Himself and keep Blake in the grip of His grace all the days of his life. *Lord Jesus, you are the Light that the darkness cannot overcome. Your Gospel and saving power have never been hindered by the times. Please save my grandson, deliver him from evil, and make him a light that shatters darkness because you are with him. Jesus, hear me now and answer with salvation and life and cause my prayers for Blake to echo beyond my brief days.*

Blake is asleep now. The floor is scattered with books, stuffed animals, and Matchbox cars—the remains of this good day. I wonder sometimes, if my life is shortened, how much will Blake remember me? Will I become just a picture in a frame and only bits of memories about birds and creeks and copperheads in shining water? I do not know what Blake will take of me into his future journey, but I know what joy he has already given me in mine.

Perhaps he will read these lines someday and know that I loved him.

*Day 91*
*April 20, 2022*

Next week I'll have the long-anticipated PET scan that will show whether the transplant succeeded in putting the cancer in remission. Sometimes I'm ready to know the outcome, but mostly I'm dreading it. These three months of waiting have been shadowed by this ominous appointment and the questions it will answer about my future days. If the scan shows there's still cancer, then my options and my days will narrow considerably.

When I was young, I always felt I had so many options in the path of life. If one thing didn't work out, no problem. There was always another option to seize, and I wasn't afraid of change. Maybe that's why I transferred colleges four times in four years but still managed to finish on time and debt-free. Life was like chess—there were a hundred ways to make the next move. However, I was no Bobby Fischer. Some decisions I made turned out to be dead ends—or worse. But God's mercy kept me from disasters, and He ordered my steps even if I was too busy or too arrogant to see it.

I was taught early, "Between the great things we cannot do and the little things we will not do lies the danger of doing nothing."[6] I never wanted to be in such danger. So I tried the navy, pastored a little country church for a time, wrote textbooks, taught history, was an advisor to a U.S. senator, and founded a mission board to serve the persecuted church. All the changes, all the options, all the possibilities fed my restless spirit. Yet I found in that mosaic of experiences that God was growing my world—and growing my view of Him, too. It was a source of tireless joy to see His glory in the faces of His children ransomed from "every tribe and language and people and nation" as I traveled to those tribes and nations to write their stories of saving grace.

But the years with their weights and losses—especially the last three years shadowed by cancer—have taken their toll on my "options." I can fully identify with something George Herbert wrote:

> When first thou didst entice to thee my heart,
>     I thought the service brave:
> So many joys I writ down for my part,
>     Besides what I might have
> Out of my stock of natural delights,
> Augmented with thy gracious benefits.
>
>             . . .
>
> At first thou gav'st me milk and sweetnesses;
>     I had my wish and way:
> My days were straw'd with flow'rs and happiness;
>     There was no month but May.
> But with my years sorrow did twist and grow,
> And made a party unawares for woe.[7]

The poem is Herbert's life story. He was distinguished at Cambridge, a member of Parliament, a pastor, and a poet without parallel. Yet tuberculosis shadowed his full, short life, claiming him at thirty-nine. I can understand Herbert's growing sense of uselessness. After "sorrow did twist and grow," he writes, "My mirth and edge was lost; a blunted knife was of more use than I."[8] Herbert closes out his poem not with a pretty bow covering his pain but instead with a plea for some little usefulness to know he had not been abandoned.

> Now I am here, what thou wilt do with me
>     None of my books will show:
> I read, and sigh, and wish I were a tree;
>     For sure I then should grow
> To fruit or shade: at least some bird would trust
> Her household to me, and I should be just. . . .
>
> Ah, my dear God! though I am clean forgot,
> Let me not love thee, if I love thee not.[9]

The last lines of the poem seem to echo Job: "Though he slay me, yet will I trust in him" (Job 13:15 KJV). That is a tenacity of faith for which I long.

I don't know why the day of the scan looms so large, but it feels like a coin toss of big consequences. On one side I see the result "You are cancer-free," which opens up time—perhaps years—and options for how to spend those gifted days.

But I also see the other side of the coin. That side of the coin reads, "There's still cancer. It's aggressive, and the transplant— the last good medical option to stop it—has failed." With that, the timetable changes, and the final chapter is shorter than we would wish. There are so many things I want to finish—and so many things I want to begin—that likely will never happen. That work will go undone. Incomplete. And my dreams will be lost in the triage of waning strength and days. Sometimes I see that side of the coin in Debbie's eyes. Something triggers it—a song, a sleepless night, a sudden memory. I don't see it every day, but still, it comes too often, as sadness takes shape, stabs her with fear, and the pain of it wells in her eyes.

All of this is what I feel—at least in my darkest moments. But what I *feel* and what I *know* are two very different things. I **know** the Good Shepherd is *good*.

> I am the good shepherd. The good shepherd lays down his life for the sheep. He who is a hired hand and not a shepherd, who does not own the sheep, sees the wolf coming and leaves the sheep and flees, and the wolf snatches them and scatters them. He flees because he is a hired hand and cares nothing for the sheep. I am the good shepherd. I know my own and my own know me, just as the Father knows me and I know the Father; and I lay down my life for the sheep.
>
> John 10:11–15

I'm struck by the word "own." Fear does not own me. Cancer does not own me. Death does not own me. My Good Shepherd owns me. By His cross He forever owns me, kept in His good hands—strong, scarred hands—that will never let go of me.

My sheep hear my voice, and I know them, and they follow me. I give them eternal life, and they will never perish, and no one will snatch them out of my hand.

John 10:27–28

I **know** my days are already numbered, regardless of the outcome of the scan.

For you formed my inward parts; you knitted me together in my mother's womb. I praise you, for I am fearfully and wonderfully made. Wonderful are your works; my soul knows it very well. My frame was not hidden from you, when I was being made in secret, intricately woven in the depths of the earth. Your eyes saw my unformed substance; in your book were written, every one of them, the days that were formed for me, when as yet there was none of them.

Psalm 139:13–16

And so, I intend to live out their number, whether few or many, to the full because I know the outcome of the next scan will not add or take away the number of days that God has in love planned for me.

I **know** life will always feel incomplete when death comes. I often think of something that John Piper wrote to me almost a year ago, and it comes to mind again tonight:

*Dear Tim,*

*As I thought about the fact that death, at almost any age, seems like an interruption that threatens to cut short things we intended to do, I thought maybe this poem I wrote for Noel on Mother's Day might encourage you.*

221

*I was building her a new bird feeder with a tall post cemented into the ground, but I did not finish it on Saturday before the Sunday of Mother's Day. Hence this poem.*

### A Sonnet for Noel on Mother's Day, 2021

For now, though almost fifty years have passed
    Since you, my love, conceived, and we would meet
Our first of five—yet even now (the last
    Well-wed) your mothering is incomplete.

Not that you have a brooding need to cling,
    But that a mother's unmet dreams deplete.
Yet even now, spent like a mountain spring,
    Your heart is full, and ev'ry longing sweet.

So I thought I would build a gift for you
    On Mother's Day, where in the morning sun
The care-free birds would eat, and you would view
    How cheerful is their toil, though never done.

And though my gift of love is incomplete,
My love is full and every longing sweet.

*May the Lord give you more years and more dispatches, and when the time of your departure comes, though all will feel incomplete, may your love be full and longings sweet.*

*John*

I always smile when I think of how my brilliant friend didn't have time to finish the bird feeder, but he had time to write a sonnet about it! But his counsel was as plain as it was kind. Death is an interruption, and so there will always be a sense of incompleteness—that's just the way of it. But God in His kindness has given us time. For some, the end comes so shockingly fast that there's no time for even a good-bye. But we've had years now. As hard as these three years have been, there has also been mercy and kindness in the giving of them.

Regardless of scan results or the number of days left in this narrowing valley, I have hope and a future because of Christ. Lord Jesus, you know, though, that my grip is weak. Yet yours is strong—and that is enough for me.

**Day 100**
**April 29, 2022**

> Two roads diverged in a wood, and I—
> I took the one less traveled by.[10]

Robert Frost's famous fork-in-the-road experience is how I feel about my cancer, which has two strains—two paths. One, anaplastic lymphocytic kinase (ALK)-positive, responds well to chemotherapy, but the more rare and more aggressive ALK-negative doesn't—and that's the kind I have. This less-traveled path is not the one I would have chosen, but here I am. And the latest scan shows that despite all the treatments, a stubborn spot of this rare blood cancer remains. And so, it likely won't be a weapon or accident that will end my life—but instead a missing molecule at the end of a genetic formula. Utterly insignificant and yet ultimately deadly.

Although the transplant did not succeed in eradicating the cancer, Dr. Chowdhury believes it did slow it down. It's still a time bomb inside of me, but perhaps it has stopped ticking for a while. She's ordered a scan in six weeks and another in three months to check if the spot is spreading. More waiting. Yet I cannot wait to live—that's a waste of time. The next scans may give me more information, but they won't give me more days. I have no illusion about how steep the way ahead will be of whatever remains of this marathon, but I'm ready to run. Or at least to walk, and then crawl—but not to sit and wait.

In Bunyan's great story, one of the pilgrims, Mr. Feeble-mind, is journeying to meet his King. Mr. Feeble-mind is beset by his many weaknesses and the dangers along the road. After a narrow escape, he shares his story with his fellow pilgrims. He is weak, but his faith is not.

> Other brunts I also look for, but this I have resolved on, to wit, to *run* when I can, to *go* when I cannot run, and to *creep* when I cannot go. As to the main, I thank him that loves me, I am fixed; my Way is before me, my mind is beyond the River that has no bridge.[11]

Debbie and I are trying to prepare ourselves for the way ahead now that we know this cancer will stay with us to the end. But so, too, will our Risen Shepherd, who has crossed "the River that has no bridge"—and then crossed it again to bring us safely over.

Our days in this journey are uneven, as is our faith. I heard courage in Debbie's voice last night as she prayed—and that gave me courage. But tonight, after the scan results were known, her voice was weighed with weariness as she lay on the bed feeling sick. We've run out of words, so I held her until the light drained from the sky: "I promise I'll stay with you as long as I can."

# ALL MY DAYS

Through many dangers, toils, and snares,
I have already come;
'Tis grace that brought me safe thus far,
And grace will lead me home.[1]

    —John Newton, "Amazing Grace"

**Artillery Road**
**October 17, 2022**

There was a time when I was not at all sure if I would live to write this chapter, but here I am on my back porch this October afternoon scribbling these lines. It's been nearly six months since I closed the previous chapter. Subsequent scans confirm that my cancer remains, but it's quiet for now. All indications are that it will likely rage whenever it resurfaces, but today is not that day. Today seems a world away from the gray light of the hospital and the IV pumps and sickening liquids slow-dripping into my veins. Instead, it's a perfect autumn afternoon—the kind that puts the O! in October. Long light and long shadows play together before dark, and the sun is brilliant to the end, touching each leaf with flame before a breeze turns some into confetti.

This last hour of day is warm enough for the back door to be left open, and the promise of supper is wafting from the kitchen to the porch. Debbie is making her justifiably famous potato soup tonight—famous to me and to all those blessed to taste it. The kitchen clatters sound like home, and I'm happy to sit and write here at my favorite perch; but I confess a pang of loss over the beauty of these irretrievable moments.

There's something in the wind this time of year that feels like an old ache. Not any wind, but a certain one. Whether it's restlessness or homesickness, I cannot say—perhaps it is both—but it's not nostalgia awakened for somewhere long ago. Instead, it's a touch of melancholy for a place I've never seen. I've felt this stirring this time of year since I was young, and I clearly recall feeling it as an early snow fell in the intensely lonely mountain pass of Lal-wa-Sarjangal. Maybe these are winds stirring through an open window high on the thin wall between here and heaven. Like so much of the rest of my wonderful life, it's a mystery to me—and some mysteries are best left in wonder.

Here in my half-acre world, the more immediate mystery is why the last hour of the day is quicker than all the rest. Already dusk's half-light has erased the trees' long shadows, and the sun is now only winking through their tousled tops. But there's still enough light to write, so at the close of this dying day, how do I pen the last lines of this book?

This story is an ordinary one. My dwindling days and diminishing strength are nothing special, since we are *all* terminal. So given that our days run swiftly toward nightfall, how do we spend them well? I have no easy answer, and I struggle with that question even as I make little plans for next week and bigger plans for next year, aware of how cancer has loosened my grip on my calendar and stripped away any illusion that I am in control of it. I've learned, though, that there's something really good about getting a proper impression of my own smallness. I've experienced this in nature while standing in a forest of sequoias, when caught in a storm at sea, and while sitting beneath the moon and stars while the sun burned off the edge of night. There's wonder in facing such immensities. I like the way the intrepid traveler Freya Stark described waiting for dawn in a faraway place: "It was still far from daylight. The high dome of heaven was revolving with peacock colors and secret constellations among the outlined rocks. . . . I sat there for over an hour, watching the moonlight retreat from the rocky bastions, a process of infinite majesty and peace."[2] In awe of her smallness before such magnificence, she was, quoting an ancient poet, "like dust in the lion's paw."[3]

It is a powerful image, for I, too, am dust, yet caught up in greater things. There are days that the fearful immensity of death looms all around me with its terrible silence and then strikes me with sorrow over this tearing of life and the pain it will leave in its wake to those I love. Yet my going to God is the glorious immensity that makes all the world's immensities of small account. And because of the resurrection, Jesus has made even the immensity of death little more than dust in the Lion's paw.

But given my apparent time crunch, is it pointless to do things I will just take to my grave? For example, is it a waste to read a book that serves no purpose except to delight with its beauty and spark my imagination? I don't think so. Is it a waste for Debbie to make potato soup tonight and dish out generous portions that will only be a memory by breakfast? I'm glad she doesn't think so! These—and many more everyday acts I could name—are part of the resistance, for we intend to defy death to the end by fully living to the end.

I know deeper shadows will fall over our happiness and will empty my chair at the table, but being frantic over how little time I have or paralyzed by fear over death are real timewasters. I want to use my time in ways that are purposeful—that is, they fulfill the purposes for which God has made me: husband, father, grandfather, friend, writer, traveler, dreamer, preacher of the Gospel. These purposes are not perfectly formed in me, but they are the broken stones in the mosaic of my life. I want my days to be brimful of life because that's why the God of all life gave them. So whether I'm reading a book, watering my garden, standing in the morning chill to listen to the early birds, or loving my wife—I think all these things make my days count as much as the more visible work that I spent my life building and doing. Over it all, I pray what Paul wrote will also be fulfilled in me: "It is my eager expectation and hope that I will not be at all ashamed, but that with full courage now as always Christ will be honored in my body, whether by life or by death" (Philippians 1:20). So I lay the offering of all my days at nail-scarred feet, knowing I'm only giving back what was never mine to keep, and in returning them, may each day have the luster of new life about it.

All along my day's journey, Christ has been my light. Even in the long hours of the darkest nights, He was the constellation of my hope and the Morning Star for whom I waited. And in this narrowing valley that my Good Shepherd has led me to and is carrying me through, His promise "I am with you" is a sacred one between us. As the old hymn says,

> The soul that on Jesus relies,
> He'll never, no never deceive;
> He freely and faithfully gives
> More blessings than we can conceive;
> Yea, down to old age he will keep,
> Nor will he forsake us at last;
> He knows, and is known by, his sheep;
> They're his, and he will hold them fast.[4]

# NOTES

1. Elisabeth Elliot, *All That Was Ever Ours* (Grand Rapids: Revell, 1988), 72.

**Readers' Guide**

1. Emily Dickinson, *Collected Poems of Emily Dickinson* (New York: Gramercy Books, 1982), 199.

2. "O Lord, My Rock and My Redeemer," music and words by Nathan Stiff. © 2017 Sovereign Grace Worship (ASCAP) (adm at IntegratedRights.com). All rights reserved. Used by permission. www.SovereignGraceMusic.org.

3. David McCullough, *Brave Companions: Portraits in History* (New York: Simon & Schuster Paperbacks, 1992), ix.

4. Ann Patchett, *These Precious Days* (New York: HarperCollins, 2021), 2.

**Dear Diary**

1. Alexander Maclaren, "Redeeming the Time," *Bible Hub*, https://bible hub.com/sermons/auth/maclaren/redeeming_the_time.htm.

2. *The Journals of Lewis and Clark*, ed. Bernard DeVoto (New York: Houghton Mifflin Company, 1997), vii.

3. Mark Helprin, "Skip the Paris Cafés and Get a Good Pen," *Wall Street Journal*, September 28, 2012, https://www.wsj.com/articles/SB10000872396390444 35880457801652082881716.

4. Alexsandr Solzhenitsyn, *Cancer Ward* (New York: Grosset and Dunlap, 1969), 445–446.

5. Georgi P. Vins, *The Gospel in Bonds* (Elkhart, IN: Russian Gospel Ministries, 1995), 9–10.

6. Simona Gorton, in personal correspondence with Tim Keesee in 2021.

**One Day to Live**

1. Robert E. Speer, *Servants of the King* (New York: Educational Department, The Board of Foreign Missions of the Presbyterian Church in the U.S.A., 1909), 99.

2. John Kelly, "Notable & Quotable: Six Seconds to Live," *The Wall Street Journal*, October 23, 2017, A15.

3. George MacDonald, *The Diary of an Old Soul* (London: Arthur C. Fifield, 1909), January 27 entry.

4. PRESENT CONCERNS by C. S. Lewis copyright © 1948 C.S. Lewis Pte. Ltd. Extract reprinted by permission.

C. S. Lewis, "On Living in an Atomic Age" (first published in 1948), *Present Concerns: Essays by C. S. Lewis*, ed. Walter Hooper (New York: Harcourt Brace Jovanovich, 1986), 73–80.

5. John Piper, "Ten Principles for Personal Productivity," April 18, 2016, Desiring God: Ask Pastor John, episode 839, https://www.desiringgod.org /interviews/ten-principles-for-personal-productivity.

6. David McCullough, *The Wright Brothers* (New York: Simon & Schuster, 2015), 109.

7. David McCullough, *The Wright Brothers*, 121.

8. J.D. Crowley, "One Day to Live," *Gospel Meditations for Missions* (Church Works Media, 2011), Day 25.

## Stumbling into the Future

1. Freya Stark, *The Journey's Echo* (New York: Harcourt, Brace & World, Inc., 1964), 54.

2. C. H. Spurgeon, *Autobiography vol. 1: The Early Years* (Carlisle, PA: The Banner of Truth Trust, 1962), 87–88.

3. Samuel M. Zwemer, *The Unoccupied Mission Fields of Africa and Asia* (New York: Student Volunteer Movement for Foreign Missions, 1911), 90.

## Time in a Rectangle

1. Janet Malcolm, *Still Pictures: On Photography and Memory* (New York: Farrar, Straus and Giroux, 2023), 39.

2. Wendell Berry, *Jayber Crow* (Berkeley, CA: Counterpoint, 2000), 24.

3. Lance Morrow, *Second Drafts of History* (New York: Basic Books, 2006), 123.

4. Frederick Buechner, *A Crazy, Holy Grace: The Healing Power of Pain and Memory* (Grand Rapids, MI: Zondervan, 2017), 58–59.

5. J. R. R. Tolkien, *The Hobbit* (New York: Houghton Mifflin Company, 1997), 287.

6. Charles Wesley, "And Can It Be, That I Should Gain?" 1738.

7. Fanny Crosby, "Blessed Assurance," 1873.

## Along the Way

1. Henry Wadsworth Longfellow, "The Arrow and the Song" in *The Book of Virtues*, ed. William J. Bennett (New York: Simon & Schuster, 1993), 341.

## In the Eye of a Storm

1. Rosaria Champagne Butterfield, *The Secret Thoughts of an Unlikely Convert* (Pittsburgh, PA: Crown & Covenant Publications, 2012), 29.

2. Butterfield, *The Secret Thoughts of an Unlikely Convert*, 21.

3. Richard Rushing, ed., *Voices from the Past: Puritan Devotional Readings* (Carlisle, PA: The Banner of Truth Trust, 2010), 159.

4. Samuel M. Zwemer, *The Glory of the Cross* (London: Marshall, Morgan, and Scott, Ltd., 1935), 34.

5. "Praise the Lord," *The Book of Psalms for Worship* (Pittsburgh, PA: Crown & Covenant, 2011), 146A. Used by permission.

6. The words *hospitality* (Romans 12:13; Hebrews 13:2; 1 Peter 4:9) and *hospitable* (1 Timothy 3:2; Titus 1:8) derive from two Greek words: *philos* (loving) and *xenos* (a stranger). They combine into one beautiful, blessed, uncomfortable word: *philoxenia* (love of strangers). This is from S. D. Renn and N. J. Sandon, eds., *Vine's Amplified Expository Dictionary of New Testament Words*, reference edition (Iowa Falls, IA: World Bible Publishers, 1991), 401.

7. Butterfield, *The Secret Thoughts of an Unlikely Convert*, 20.

8. Rosaria Butterfield, *The Gospel Comes with a House Key* (Wheaton, IL: Crossway, 2018), 41.

9. "Hear, O Hear Us," *The Book of Psalms for Worship* (Pittsburgh, PA: Crown & Covenant, 2011), 80. Used by permission.

10. "Hear, O Hear Us," *The Book of Psalms for Worship*, 80. Used by permission.

11. Rosaria Butterfield, "Can the Pandemic Be an Answered Prayer?" Desiring God, May 23, 2020, https://www.desiringgod.org/articles/can-the-pandemic-be-an-answered-prayer.

12. "O Let Your Lovingkindnesses Now Come," *The Book of Psalms for Worship* (Pittsburgh, PA: Crown & Covenant, 2011), 119F. Used by permission.

13. THE LION, THE WITCH AND THE WARDROBE by C. S. Lewis copyright © 1950 C. S. Lewis Pte. Ltd. Extract reprinted by permission. C. S. Lewis, *The Lion, the Witch, and the Wardrobe* (New York: Harper Trophy, 2000), 80.

## Day of Hopeful Planting

1. John Bunyan, *The Pilgrim's Progress* (1678: Edinburgh: Banner of Truth, 1979), 376.

2. Bunyan, *The Pilgrim's Progress*, 377.

3. George Herbert, "The Dawning," *The Complete English Works* (London: Random House, 1995), 108–109.

4. Wendell Berry, "The Plan," from *New Collected Poems*. © 1964, 1968 by Wendell Berry. Reprinted with the permission of The Permissions Company, LLC, on behalf of Counterpoint Press, counterpointpress.com.

5. I'd also like to share another quote from Ken and Joni's struggle during that time:

Joni suddenly remembered something Alan Redpath, a British pastor and author, had written. "Remember what Redpath said, Ken? I think I can quote it. 'There is no circumstance, no trouble, no testing, that can ever touch me until, first of all, it has gone past God and past Christ, right through to me. If it has come *that* far, it has come with great purpose.' Ken, I believe this cancer has come with great purpose."

Ken and Joni Eareckson Tada, *Joni & Ken: An Untold Love Story* (Grand Rapids, MI: Zondervan, 2013), 24.

6. Ken and Joni Eareckson Tada, *Joni & Ken: An Untold Love Story*, 21.

7. Charles Spurgeon, "The Friend of God," from Metropolitan Tabernacle Pulpit Volume 33, The Spurgeon Center, May 8, 1887, https://www.spurgeon.org/collection/metropolitan-tabernacle-pulpit-volume-33/.

8. John 10:27–30.

## Knee-Deep in Wonders

1. Quoted in Joni Eareckson Tada, *A Place of Healing* (Colorado Springs, CO: David C. Cook, 2010), 111.

2. David McCullough, *Brave Companions*, 25.

3. McCullough, *Brave Companions*, 25.

4. THE MAGICIAN'S NEPHEW by C. S. Lewis copyright © 1955 C. S. Lewis Pte. Ltd. Extract reprinted by permission.

C. S. Lewis, *The Chronicles of Narnia Book One: The Magician's Nephew* (New York: Harper Trophy, 2000), 112.

5. James Whitcomb Riley, "Knee-deep in June," *The World's Best Poetry, Volume V*, ed. Bliss Carman et al., (Philadelphia: John D. Morris & Co., 1904), www.bartleby.com/360/5/80.html.

6. Julie Zickefoose, "'An Immense World' Review: Where Beasts Have Us Beat," *The Wall Street Journal*, June 17, 2022, https://www.wsj.com/articles/an-immense-world-book-review-where-beasts-have-us-beat-11655481384.

## The Day the Walls Came Down

1. Robert Frost, "Mending Wall," *The Poetry of Robert Frost*, ed. Edward Connery Lathem (New York: Holt, Rinehart and Winston, 1969), 34.

2. Norman P. Grubb, *C. T. Studd: Cricketer and Pioneer* (Fort Washington, PA: CLC Publications, 2008), 145.

3. Ioannis Mantzikos, "The Greek Gateway to Jihad," *CTC Sentinel*, June 2016, Volume 9, Issue 6, 16–18.

4. John Bunyan, *Grace Abounding to the Chief of Sinners* (London: The Religious Tract Society, 1905), 13.

## Brave Music

1. Edmond Budry, trans. Richard B. Hoyle, "Thine Is the Glory," 1923.
2. Joni Eareckson Tada, in a personal note, January 22, 2022.
3. Zoom call with Joni Eareckson Tada on November 29, 2021.
4. Fanny Crosby, "All the Way My Savior Leads Me," 1875.
5. Jean Sophia Pigott, "Jesus, I Am Resting, Resting," 1876.
6. Augustus M. Toplady, "Rock of Ages," 1776.
7. P. P. Bliss, "'Man of Sorrows' What a Name," 1875.

## The Sweet Psalmist of Texas

1. Andrew Peterson, *Adorning the Dark* (Nashville, TN: B&H Publishing, 2019), 40.
2. "Wake Up," music and words by Caroline Cobb Smith. ©2013 Sing the Story Music (ASCAP) (adm at IntegratedRights.com). All rights reserved. Used by permission. www.CarolineCobb.com.
3. "Tell That Story," music and words by Caroline Cobb Smith. ©2019 Sing the Story Music (ASCAP). All rights reserved. Used by permission. www.CarolineCobb.com.
4. "Psalm 91 (My Refuge and My Fortress)," music and words by Caroline Cobb Smith. © 2022 Sing the Story Music (ASCAP) (adm at IntegratedRights.com). All rights reserved. Used by permission. www.CarolineCobb.com.
5. "Psalm 63 (Better Than Life)," music and words by Caroline Cobb Smith © 2022 Sing the Story Music (ASCAP) (adm at IntegratedRights.com). All rights reserved. Used by permission. www.CarolineCobb.com.
6. "Psalm 119 (I Love Your Word)," music and words by Caroline Cobb Smith and Anne-Claire Cummings. © 2022 Anne Claire Cummings (ASCAP) and Sing the Story Music (ASCAP) (adm at IntegratedRights.com). All rights reserved. Used by permission. www.CarolineCobb.com. www.Anne-Claire Cummings.com.
7. "Psalm 91 (My Refuge and My Fortress)," music and words by Caroline Cobb Smith. © 2022 Sing the Story Music (ASCAP) (adm at Integrated Rights.com). All rights reserved. Used by permission. www.CarolineCobb.com.

## Five Witnesses

1. Elisabeth Elliot, *A Path Through Suffering* (Grand Rapids, MI: Revell, 1990), 121.
2. Anonymous, "The Power of His Rising" (harmonization copyright Fred and Ruth Coleman, 2013). Used with permission.
3. Robert D. Kaplan, *Soldiers of God: With the Mujahidin in Afghanistan* (Boston: Houghton Mifflin Company, 1990), 49.
4. Cheryl Beckett song based on Isaiah 43.

## Another Way to Die

1. "Out of the Depths," music and words by Bob Kauflin. © 2008 Sovereign Grace Praise (BMI) (adm at IntegratedRights.com). All rights reserved. Used by permission. www.SovereignGraceMusic.org.

2. Charles H. Spurgeon, *Beside Still Waters: Words of Comfort for the Soul*, ed. Roy H. Clarke (Nashville: Thomas Nelson Inc., 1999), 2.

## In Habakkuk's Tower

1. John Piper, *When the Darkness Will Not Lift* (Nottingham, England: Inter-Varsity Press, 2007), 37.

2. Wendell Berry, excerpt from "The Meadow," from *New Collected Poems*. © 1964, 1968 by Wendell Berry. Reprinted with the permission of The Permissions Company, LLC, on behalf of Counterpoint Press, counterpoint press.com.

3. César Malan (trans. George W. Bethune), "It Is Not Death to Die," 1847.

4. Bunyan, *The Pilgrim's Progress*, 181–182.

5. Tim Keller, *Making Sense of God: An Invitation to the Skeptical* (New York: Viking, 2016), 166.

6. Dylan Thomas, *In Country Sleep, and Other Poems* (London: Dent, 1952), 19.

7. Charles Spurgeon, *Metropolitan Tabernacle Pulpit*, Volume 20, 1874 (Pasadena, TX: Pilgrim Publications, 1986), 223.

8. George Herbert, *The Complete English Works* (London: David Campbell Publishers Ltd., 1995), 165.

9. Andrew Peterson, "Hosanna," *Resurrection Letters Vol II* (Centricity Music, 2008).

## Chemo Days

1. Robert Frost, "Dust of Snow," *The Poetry of Robert Frost*, ed. Edward Connery Lathem, 221.

2. Robert Lowry, "How Can I Keep from Singing?" 1869.

3. Michael Collins, *Carrying the Fire: An Astronaut's Journeys* (New York: Farrar, Straus and Giroux, 1989), 352–353.

4. Grant Gordon, ed., *Wise Counsel: John Newton's Letters to John Ryland, Jr.* (Edinburgh: The Banner of Truth Trust, 2009), 165.

5. Gordon, *Wise Counsel*, 164

6. Robert Frost, "The November Guest," *The Poetry of Robert Frost*, ed. Edward Connery Lathem, 6–7.

7. Gloria Furman, "The Global Rhythm of Prayer and Praise," October 25, 2014, http://www.gloriafurman.com/blog/2014/10/the-global-rhythm-of -prayer-and-praise.

8. Elvina M. Hall, "Jesus Paid It All," 1865.

## Christmas Day

1. Laura Ingalls Wilder, *Little House on the Prairie* (New York: Harper & Row, 1953), 250.

2. George Herbert, "The Dawning," *The Complete English Works* (London: Random House, 1995), 108.

## Numbered Days

1. Elisabeth Elliot, *These Strange Ashes: Is God Still in Charge?* (Grand Rapids, MI: Revell, 2004), 146–147.

2. Attributed to Rev. John McNeill in personal correspondence with Joni Eareckson Tada.

3. J. R. R. Tolkien, *The Two Towers* (Boston: Houghton Mifflin Company, 2002), 520.

4. Stanislaw Baranczak, "If China," *Against Forgetting: Twentieth-Century Poetry of Witness*, ed. Carolyn Forché (W.W. Norton & Company, 1993), 480.

5. John Burroughs, "The Bluebird," *Harper's Magazine*, June 1903.

6. Often attributed to Adolphe-Louis-Frédéric-Théodore Monod (1802–1856).

7. George Herbert, "Affliction 1," *The Complete English Works* (New York: Alfred A. Knopf, 1995), 44.

8. Herbert, "Affliction 1," 45.

9. Herbert, "Affliction 1," 46.

10. Robert Frost, "The Road Not Taken," *The Poetry of Robert Frost*, ed. Edward Connery Lathem, 105.

11. Bunyan, *The Pilgrim's Progress*, 322.

## All My Days

1. John Newton, "Amazing Grace," 1779.

2. Freya Stark, *The Valleys of the Assassins*, quoted in Paul Theroux, *The Tao of Travel: Enlightenments from Lives on the Road* (New York: Houghton Mifflin Harcourt, 2011), 237.

3. Stark, *The Valleys of the Assassins*, quoted in Theroux, *The Tao of Travel*, 237.

4. W. Gadsby, "Poor Sinner, Dejected with Fear," 1844.

**Tim Keesee** is the founder and executive director of Frontline Missions International (FMI), an organization that, for over thirty years, has served to advance the Gospel in the world's difficult places. In that capacity, he has traveled to over a hundred countries, reporting on the Church from the former Iron Curtain countries to war-torn Bosnia, Iraq, and Afghanistan. Tim is also the executive producer of the *Dispatches from the Front* film series, which highlights the marvelous extent, diversity, and unity of Christ's Kingdom in our world. He and his wife, Debbie, have two married children and one grandson.